Coping Strategies to Promote Mental Health

This manual offers care providers a unique combination of evidence-based methods for adult learning and coping strategy development when training clients individually or in groups.

Coping strategies help clients to engage and thrive in meaningful self-care, as well as productive and leisure occupations. The coping strategies are divided into four categories: health and wellness routines, changing the body's response to stress, changing the situation, and changing attitudes. Each category contains four modules with client handouts for coping strategy training, including sleep hygiene, suicide safety planning, setting healthy boundaries, and cultivating gratitude. Every module contains a facilitator lesson plan, specific learning outcomes, and examples of expected client responses to ensure the learning is taking place.

Occupational therapists and other care providers, both novice and experienced, will find this manual useful to improve efficiencies in practice and provision of meaningful teachings.

Theresa Straathof, OT Reg. (Ont.), is an occupational therapist at The Ottawa Hospital in Ontario, Canada with 30 years of practice. Special interests include coping strategy training and suicide prevention.

"Once again, Theresa has shared her depth of knowledge and practical strategies in an accessible way for occupational therapists at all levels of their practice. Having used the first manual, *Coping Strategies to Promote Occupational Engagement and Recovery* (McNamara & Straathof, 2017*)*, for several years in our practice, our group of occupational therapists is excited to see this next volume with even more relevant, useful guides for group and individual coping session delivery. The handouts are easy for occupational therapists to sort and select, and easy for clients to read and understand; a recipe for success across many clinical environments."

Fiona Smith Bradley, OT Reg, *occupational therapist, partner, Modern OT, Ottawa, ON*

"An excellent follow-through from the first book. The modules are well thought out and beautifully presented. A very potent tool box for Mental Health in-patients and for Day Hospitals. Easily adaptable to individual therapy. The suicide prevention and anger management modules alone are worth the cover price."

Keith Anderson, MD, FRCP(C)

"The step wise approach based on adult learning principles makes this book extremely easy to refer to, to use with clients and guarantees benefits for them, as it always leads to identifiable and observable changes in behaviours. The links made between cognitive-behavioural principles and various occupational therapy concepts brings an innovative aspect to client care and gives a very unique OT lens to the book. The handouts are user friendly, well done and straight to the point. They are clear, concrete, and link to meaningful behavior change and participation-based examples. This book will be a very useful resource for occupational therapists working in adult mental health and community-based workers needing resources for people with severe mental illness."

Suzanne Rouleau, OT, MSc, *occupational therapist-psychotherapist, assistant-professor, Occupational Therapy program, McGill University*

"Theresa's book is an invaluable resource for Occupational Therapists and other care providers. It provides clear and practical modules, including learning plans and activities, covering many key coping strategies. Theresa's modules have become an integral part of the treatment for many of my patients as they strive for improved mental health and wellness."

Gary Kay, MD, FRCPC, *staff psychiatrist and inpatient director, The Ottawa Hospital, Civic Campus*

"This book is an essential expansion from the previous *Coping Strategies to Promote Occupational Engagement and Recovery: A Program Manual for Occupational Therapists and Other Care Providers*. The modules' structure makes the content accessible to care providers regardless of experience level. The details help to build the care provider's confidence and enables pre-application preparation. I have found that the functional real-life examples are relatable to clients from diverse backgrounds, and with cultural humility can be applied to a variety of contexts. In my previous work as a mental health nurse in a remote Northern Indigenous community I used the modules daily. I received feedback that the worksheets were valuable, often-referenced takeaways. The practical modules in this book successfully translate abstract concepts into actionable, client-centred plans. I look forward to using this book in future practice and am sure it will be an indispensable resource for many care providers."

Marley Pickles White, RN

Coping Strategies to Promote Mental Health

Training Modules for Occupational Therapists
and Other Care Providers

Theresa Straathof

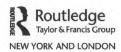

NEW YORK AND LONDON

First published 2022
by Routledge
605 Third Avenue, New York, NY 10158

and by Routledge
2 Park Square, Milton Park, Abingdon, Oxon OX14 4RN

Routledge is an imprint of the Taylor & Francis Group, an informa business

Library of Congress Cataloging-in-Publication Data
Names: Straathof, Theresa, author.
Title: Coping strategies to promote mental health: training modules for occupational therapists and other care providers / Theresa Straathof.
Description: New York, NY: Routledge, 2022. |
Includes bibliographical references and index.
Identifiers: LCCN 2021015153 (print) | LCCN 2021015154 (ebook) |
ISBN 9781032039176 (hardback) | ISBN 9781032039169 (paperback) |
ISBN 9781003189695 (ebook)
Subjects: LCSH: Mental health services. |
Mental health promotion. | Mental health planning.
Classification: LCC RA790.5 .S76 2022 (print) |
LCC RA790.5 (ebook) | DDC 362.2–dc23
LC record available at https://lccn.loc.gov/2021015153
LC ebook record available at https://lccn.loc.gov/2021015154

ISBN: 978-1-032-03917-6 (hbk)
ISBN: 978-1-032-03916-9 (pbk)
ISBN: 978-1-003-18969-5 (ebk)

DOI: 10.4324/9781003189695

Typeset in Times New Roman
by Newgen Publishing UK

For my father, my role model for perseverance.

Contents

List of Handouts

- Sleep hygiene checklist
- Sleep facts
- Card game: Answer sheet
- My four chosen behaviours to improve sleep quality
- One-day schedule
- Challenges impacting medication adherence
- Possible solutions to improve medication adherence
- Recipe for daily health
- Strategies for forming habits
- My plan to form a health habit
- Strategies to simplify meal preparation
- Obstacles and solutions for meal preparation
- One-day menu
- Examples of barriers and strategies for making change
- Action plan for change
- Expanding my community network
- Boundaries versus walls
- Defining boundaries
- Personal scenario
- Is this a boundary violation?
- Tips for setting boundaries
- Personal rules for boundaries
- Behaviour experiment
- Getting unstuck
- Overcoming avoidance
- Action initiative
- Game template and resource for therapist/facilitator
- Anger game: Answers
- Strategies for changing thoughts, behaviours and physical symptoms of anger
- Anger management plan

- Activities with a sensory focus
- Emotional first aid: Items and actions
- Rating tool for mood levels
- My first aid kit for emotional comfort
- Suicide safety plan for occupational engagement and recovery (SSP-OEAR) – sample
- Suicide safety plan for occupational engagement and recovery (SSP-OEAR)
- Mini suicide safety plan – wallet-size cards
- Accessing your strengths
- Matching exercise (Max)
- Using strengths to develop resilience
- Symbol of strength
- Steps to creative problem solving
- Problem solving worksheet
- Key factors in building resilience, wellness and happiness
- Occupation categories for resilience, wellness and happiness
- Case scenario: Amara
- Sample gratitude journal: Amara
- Mix and match: Gratitude
- Mix and match: Gratitude answer sheet
- Gratitude journal

Author Biography

Theresa Straathof practices as an occupational therapist in acute mental health at The Ottawa Hospital. She has presented nationally and internationally on topics for behaviour activation, adult learning, coping strategy training and suicide safety planning. She is an active member with the Canadian Association of Occupational Therapists' practice network – Addressing Suicide in Occupational Therapy Practice. Her first book, *Coping Strategies to Promote Occupational Engagement and Recovery* has sold internationally and proved useful in remote northern communities and a variety of health care settings.

She holds a degree in Occupational Therapy from Western University and a diploma in adult education from St. Francis Xavier University.

Acknowledgements

I would like to express my gratitude to the many who have helped with the bringing together of this book:

To the clients I work with, who demonstrate remarkable resilience, a desire to persevere in the face of challenge, and provide willingness to engage in learning.

To my colleagues at The Ottawa Hospital past and present, both in occupational therapy and on the acute mental health unit, who offer encouragement, advocate for the benefits of occupational therapy, and provide protected time and space to run these training sessions.

To the student occupational therapists that provide insight and feedback for improving the modules. Special recognition goes to Émilie Isabelle Cousineau and Marie-Laurence Lambert who provided research support for the suicide safety and meal simplification modules, respectfully.

To my colleagues at the Canadian Association of Occupational Therapists who provide opportunities for networking with colleagues and dissemination of coping strategy resources.

To the professional staff at St. Francis Xavier University Adult Education Faculty for their diploma program that set the foundation for this important work to be passed on to others.

To Routledge and Taylor & Francis Group for supporting this endeavor and for their guidance in bringing this work to completion.

To my longtime mentor and friend, Mary McNamara. Her desire for program improvement and evidence-based practice is infectious, and is the catalyst on my own journey towards excellence in adult education.

To my husband Chris who always provides a listening ear and encouragement to push further with my many projects, and my three children who make me proud and grateful every day.

Thank you

Introduction

Theresa Straathof

Introduction

A core belief of occupational therapy is that the person derives a sense of purpose and connection through meaningful occupations in the domains of self-care, productivity and leisure. Coping strategies empower clients to engage in these occupations and to seek balance amongst the three domains. This book provides modules for professionals to train adult clients in coping strategies. The client applies the learning to real life problems related to what they need and want to do.

The book modules follow the collaborative approach first outlined in: *Coping Strategies to Promote Occupational Engagement and Recovery: A Program Manual for Occupational Therapists and Other Care Providers* (McNamara & Straathof, 2017), which provides details of the foundational models in occupational therapy, adult learning, learning evaluation and recovery. It also includes evidence that supports the teaching process and the coping content used in the modules. The modules in this book expand on evidence-based coping content for promoting wellness and resilience, such as sleep hygiene, suicide safety planning, setting healthy boundaries and gratitude, etc. Interesting methods are used to teach the content including games, case studies, checklists, experiments, mix/match exercises and journaling. The modules need not be offered in the sequence they appear. Instead, the facilitator can choose what training topics are suitable based on an assessment of the client's needs. A brief overview follows for coping categories, training process for adult learning and the modules.

Four Coping Categories

There are four categories of coping strategies, each bringing something unique to managing personal health and building resilience: a) Health and wellness routines; b) Changing the situation; c) Changing the body response and d) Changing attitude (Straathof, Simoneau & McNamara, 2019; Tubesing & Tubesing, 1983). Healthy routines reduce physical and mental stress by adding structure and predictability to

DOI: 10.4324/9781003189695-1

daily activity. Changing situations through actions like setting goals, assertive communication and time management return a sense of control to the circumstances. Changing the body's physical symptoms and emotional distress is important to override the fight, flight or freeze response, so that reasoning and problem solving can occur. Changing attitudes, perceptions or negative thoughts to be positive, compassionate or accepting can reduce intense emotions. The modules in this manual relate to content from these four categories.

Training Process for Adult Learning

> Please note that "learners" is the term used by Kolb in his work, while "client" is the term used by occupational therapists when referring to those individuals they work with. The term "learner" is used in the modules as it follows Kolb's process.

The training process for each module incorporates principles of adult learning (Knowles, 1989), and an Adult Learning Model (ALM) as introduced by Kolb (2014) and expanded upon by Saint Francis Xavier University (2017). Learning is evaluated before the learner leaves the session to facilitate learning transfer to personal environments (Kirkpatrick & Kirkpatrick, 2006). Kolb's learning cycle is where the actual learning takes place and includes the four stages: Experience, reflection, generalization and application. Questions and activities help move the learner through the cycle.

Experience includes information that captures the attention and senses of the learner. It could include activities like handouts, demonstrations, or lecture, etc. Reflection taps into the learner's recall of and emotional reaction to the experience. This stage provides opportunity for the facilitator to review important information from the experience that the learner may not have focused on. It also allows opportunity to acknowledge the learner's feelings and provide validation and reassurance as appropriate. Generalization allows the learner to find relevance and meaning in the new information, and to consider challenges or benefits of applying the learning. At this stage, the facilitator may also provide a top-up of information. Application allows the learner to try out a part of the learning or to make a plan to use the learning.

The set up for each module with explanation of the 14 steps follows.

1. Learning point: A brief synopsis of the learning concept that is the focus of the session to guide the learning design.
2. Learning objective: A clear and concrete description of what action the client displays at the end of the session. Objectives relate to domains of learning for

new knowledge, skill or affect. Knowledge tests the understanding of concepts, skills test performance and affect relates to a shift in attitude or buy in to using the new learning.

Learning objectives have four components. First, the condition outlines activities or resources in the learning session. Second, the performance statement clarifies what the learner will do. Third, the standard outlines how well the performance statement is done. Finally, the evaluators are named as they will determine if the standard of learning is met.

3. Materials: A list of items needed for the session, some of which need to be prepared before the session begins.

4. Handouts: A list of the resource handouts for the facilitator and those handouts for client use.

5. Orientation: A brief overview of the coping strategy that will be taught to provide context and relevance to the learner. This is the first step in the learning where the learner is present.

6. Clarification: An outline of the agenda so that learners know what to expect and what will be asked of them during the session.

7. Warm-up: An activity that engages participation from the learners to assist in forming the group and getting to know each other. The activity relates to the session theme.

8. Experience: An activity that provides sensory information and captures the interest of the learner.

9. Reflection: An invitation to the learner to provide information on what was noticed or their emotional reaction to the experience.

10. Generalization: An opportunity for higher levels of thinking through the learner's abstraction of concepts and finding significance or meaning in the learning.

11. Application: A chance for the learner to try out techniques or make a plan to use the new learning in real life.

12. Evaluation of the learning objective: An action from the learner within the session, measuring success of the original learning objective. The learner connects the learning to personal and meaningful occupations in self-care, productivity or leisure. If the objective is learned in the session, it stands to reason that transfer of learning outside of the session is then possible.

13. Wrap up: A time set aside to answer final questions and thank learners for participating.

14. References for module and handouts: A list of sources for the evidence that supports the coping strategy content from the session.

The Modules

The modules are set up to run in a group format for 60-minute sessions. The modules can easily be adapted to one-to-one sessions, and this is the preferred method for the suicide safety planning module. What is imperative to the learning is to follow the process model and structure. Questions and actions, as well as suggestions for expected learner responses provide guidance for the facilitator but can be modified to suit the learner's needs, the environment and the time for completion. Where case scenarios are included, the names and circumstances have been altered to protect confidentiality.

The modules in the health and wellness section focus on sleep hygiene, medication adherence, forming healthy habits and simplification of meals, as related to integrating health actions into daily routines.

The modules for changing the situation relate to goal setting and forming healthy relationships. Topics include overcoming roadblocks to change and setting goals, increasing support networks through building community resources, and defining and setting healthy boundaries.

The modules to change the body response to stress focus on behaviour activation, managing anger, distress tolerance and suicide safety planning. Behaviour activation strategies move clients from avoidance to doing. The remaining modules focus on regulation of emotions. The benefit of making a suicide safety plan is that in a crisis, the plan of constructive action is already established and therefore may be easier to carry out.

The modules for changing attitude explore positive thinking, gratitude or personal strengths. A technique to structure problem solving is also outlined.

Conclusion

The structure of training supports even the novice practitioner to provide meaningful and collaborative coping strategy teachings. Efficiencies occur because of the learning design, the evaluation of actual learning, and having handouts readily available. These coping strategy modules provide the client with concrete practice to improve occupational possibilities in their lives.

For an enhanced understanding of the concepts referred to in this book, please refer to *Coping Strategies to Promote Occupational Engagement and Recovery: A Program Manual for Occupational Therapists and Other Care Providers* (McNamara & Straathof, 2017). There you will also find tips to design new modules, illustration of module uses through case examples and 30 additional modules and handouts for goal setting, healthy lifestyles, stress management, assertive communication, self-esteem and shifting attitude. The module layout design is adapted and reprinted with the permission of CAOT Publications ACE and St. Francis Xavier University. The small three-circle design on the handouts represent the three components of occupation: Self-care, productivity and leisure. There is a significant relationship between use of coping strategies and successful engagement in meaningful occupation. The design is reprinted with permission from CAOT Publications ACE.

References

Kirkpatrick, D., & Kirkpatrick, J. (2006). *Evaluating Training Programs: Third edition.* San Francisco, CA: Berrett-Koehler Publishers, Inc.

Knowles, M. S. (1989). *The Making of an Adult Educator*. San Francisco, CA: Jossey-Bass Inc.

Kolb, D. A. (2014). *Experiential Learning: Experience as the source of learning and development* (2nd ed.). Englewood Cliffs, NJ: Prentice-Hall.

McNamara, M., & Straathof, T. (2017). *Coping strategies to promote occupational engagement and recovery: A program manual for occupational therapists and other care providers.* Ottawa, Ontario: CAOT.

St. Francis Xavier University. (2017). *Diploma in Adult Education.* Retrieved from: www2.mystfx.ca/adult-education-diploma/.

Straathof, T., Simoneau, E., & McNamara, M. (2019). Occupational therapy in acute mental health: Proposal for practice. *Occupational Therapy Now,* 21, 14–16.

Tubesing, N., & Tubesing, D. (eds). (1983). *Structured Exercises in Stress Management* (Vol. 1). Duluth, MN: Whole Person Associates.

1 Modules

Health and Wellness Routines

1.1 Sleep Hygiene to Improve Daily Occupations

LEARNING POINT

How one prepares for sleep can influence the quality of rest achieved.

LEARNING OBJECTIVE

Given checklist, sleep hygiene game, lecture, discussion, practice and feedback;

The learner will value sleep hygiene;

To the extent that at least four behaviours to promote healthy sleep are chosen from guidelines, and then are written in a schedule on provided template, and a verbal commitment is made to follow one named behaviour for two days;

As evaluated by self, peers and therapist/facilitator.

MATERIALS

Whiteboard or flipchart and markers, cards for sleep game (copied from handout: Card game: Answer sheet, cut and shuffled)

DOI: 10.4324/9781003189695-2

HANDOUTS

- Sleep hygiene checklist
- Sleep facts
- Card game: Answer sheet
- My four chosen behaviours to improve sleep quality
- One-day schedule

Table 1.1 Sleep hygiene to improve daily occupations

Time frame	Learning stage	Facilitator	Expected learner response
2 minutes	Orientation	[Say] Welcome, etc. [Say] Quality of sleep can be determined by how one prepares for sleep. Factors related to sleep hygiene, environment, relaxation and managing thoughts might improve deep, restful sleep and wellness (Mass & Robbins, 2012).	
3 minutes	Clarification	[Say] The objective is: To schedule behaviours for improving sleep. [Say] Today we will: • Complete a self-assessment of factors to improve sleep • Review sleep facts • Carry out a quiz on healthy and unhealthy sleep habits	

(continued)

Table 1.1 Cont.

Time frame	Learning stage	Facilitator	Expected learner response
		• Map four behaviours in our daily routine to improve sleep • Make a commitment to participate in these routines [Ask] Are we good to go?	Yes.
5 minutes	Warm-up	[Say] Let's consider things that might improve sleep quality. The first person will say their name, followed by … "I went to the store to buy …," then list something that might improve sleep. The next person will start with the same sentence and include what the first person said plus one new item. For example, I went to the store to buy a relaxation tape. We will continue until everyone has one or two turns.	Examples could include: Decaf coffee, herbal tea, eye mask, affirmation booklet, alarm clock, walking shoes, dark curtains, etc.
7 minutes	Experience	[Do] Provide handout: **Sleep hygiene checklist.** [Say] This checklist includes tips that can improve quality of sleep. For each tip, rate if you do this rarely, sometimes or regularly.	Each member completes the checklist individually.

8 minutes	Reflection	[Ask] Did any tips that were suggested surprise you? What was a personal area of strength? What may need improvement? How do you feel when you see the number of tips you already use?	Yes – likely Personal responses. Perhaps surprised, encouraged.
12 minutes	Generalization	[Ask] What keeps us from using good sleep practices for quality rest? [Do] Provide handout: **Sleep facts.** [Say] Here are some sleep facts based on research literature and specialists on sleep quality. I will read them out loud. [Ask] Which one fact may be impacting your quality of sleep lately?	Lack of knowledge of strategies or false beliefs of things to improve sleep such as alcohol use. Lack of skills (e.g. reframing worry thoughts, relaxation techniques). Decreased value placed on practicing effective sleep tips. Personal response.

(continued)

Table 1.1 Cont.

Time frame	Learning stage	Facilitator	Expected learner response
10 minutes	Application	[Do] Distribute cards for sleep game quiz. Divide learners into two teams and provide each team with half of the cards, ensuring each has an assortment of healthy and unhealthy habits. [Say] Each team will take turns reading a card from the pile out loud. The other team will be given a point if they can correctly identify the idea as a healthy or unhealthy factor for quality of sleep. A second point will be provided if that same team can explain why it is healthy or unhealthy. I will keep score. (Optional) A third point will be provided if the team can provide a healthy alternative for an unhealthy habit. [Do] Refer to handout: **Card game: Answer sheet** to assist with discussion. Provide this handout on completion of the game to all learners.	Learners take turns playing game.

12 minutes	Evaluation	[Do] Provide handout: **My four chosen behaviours to improve sleep quality** and handout: **One-day schedule.** [Say] Choose four behaviours from the checklist completed earlier in the group that you will use to promote sleep quality. Define your actions to support the behaviour. Map them on your one-day schedule. [Say] With a peer, share behaviour that you are committed to doing for the next two days to improve sleep.	Given checklist, sleep hygiene game, lecture, discussion, practice and feedback; The learner will value sleep hygiene; To the extent that at least four behaviours to promote healthy sleep are chosen from guidelines, and then are written in a schedule on provided template, and a verbal commitment is made to follow one named behaviour for two days; As evaluated by self, peers and therapist/facilitator.
1 minute	Wrap up	[Ask] Are there any questions? [Do] Thank everyone for coming and participating.	Personal response.

Reference

Mass, J., & Robbins, R. (2012). *Sleep for success! Everything you must know about sleep but are too tired to ask.* Authorhouse: Indiana.

References for Handouts

Fung, C., Wiseman-Hakes, C., Stergiou-Kita, M., Nguyen, M., & Colantonio, A. (2013). Time to wake up: Bridging the gap between theory and practice for sleep in occupational therapy. *British Journal of Occupational Therapy.* 76/8. 384–386. https://doi.org/10.4276%2F030802213X13757040168432

Garett, R., Liu, S., & Young, S. (2016). The relationship between social media use and sleep quality among undergraduate students. *Information, Communication & Society.* 21:2 163–173. https://doi.org/10.1080/1369118X.2016.1266374

Jacobus, J., Bava, S., Cohen-Zion, M., Mahmood, O., & Tapert, S. (2009). Functional consequences of marijuana use in adolescents. *Pharmacology Biochemistry Behaviour.* 92(4). 559–565. doi: 10.1016/j.pbb.2009.04.001

Mass, J., & Robbins, R. (2012). *Sleep for success! Everything you must know about sleep but are too tired to ask.* Authorhouse: Indiana.

Peach, H., Gaultney, J., & Gray, D. (2016). Sleep hygiene and sleep quality as predictors of positive and negative dimensions of mental health in college students. *Cogent Psychology.* 3(1). https://doi.org/10.1080/23311908.2016.1168768

1.2 Medication Adherence as Part of a Healthy Routine

LEARNING POINT

Medication adherence is an important part of treatment success.

LEARNING OBJECTIVE

Given lecture, discussion, practice and feedback;

The learner will commit to medication adherence;

To the extent that three strategies are named;

As evaluated by self, peers and therapist/facilitator.

MATERIALS

Whiteboard or flipchart and markers

HANDOUTS

- Challenges impacting medication adherence
- Possible solutions to improve medication adherence

Table 1.2 Medication adherence as part of a healthy routine

Time frame	Learning stage	Facilitator	Expected learner response
2 minutes	Orientation	[Say] Welcome, etc. [Say] An important part of recovery is taking medications as prescribed, yet there can be many barriers to doing so. The consequences of not taking or stopping medication can include a risk of relapse, increase hospitalizations, worsening of disease and increased health care costs (Jimmy & Jose, 2011).	
3 minutes	Clarification	[Say] The objective is: To name three strategies for medication adherence. [Say] Today we will: • Differentiate between medication compliance and adherence • Brainstorm barriers to medication adherence • Identify strategies for adherence • Make a plan to implement one strategy today [Ask] Are we good to go?	Yes.

5 minutes	Warm-up	[Say] There is a difference between medication compliance and adherence. Compliance is following your doctor's instruction based on their position of authority. Adherence means you and the doctor consider expert medical opinion and what is important to you (Jimmy & Jose, 2011).
		Examples of information: I work the night shift and cannot be sleepy from medication, I have a hard time remembering to take medication, etc.
		Please suggest questions to ask or information to share with a doctor that might improve medication adherence. For example: Asking the doctor what to do if a dose of medication is forgotten. Do you take it as soon as you remember or wait for the next dose time?
		Examples of questions: What are the side effects? How long will I need to take it? Is there a cost? etc.
7 minutes	Experience	[Do] Provide handout: **Challenges impacting medication adherence and highlighters.**
		[Say] There are reasons for medication non-adherence. Let's read the handout and then you will be invited to check off any reasons that may be a factor for you.	Learners complete handout individually.
10 minutes	Reflection	[Ask] What did you notice?	Examples: Perhaps one reason only, perhaps several reasons.
		Did any reasons seem familiar to you?	Likely yes.

(continued)

Table 1.2 Cont.

Time frame	Learning stage	Facilitator	Expected learner response
12 minutes	Generalization	[Ask] What barriers do you face in medication adherence and why? What would be a benefit for you if you could find a solution to the barrier? Why?	Personal responses.
10 minutes	Application	[Do] Provide handout: **Possible solutions to improve medication adherence.** [Say] Let's look at possible solutions to improve medication adherence. Choose two strategies that may be helpful for you.	Learners complete handout individually.
10 minutes	Evaluation	[Say] Putting an alarm on your phone, or questioning your doctor about your medication could help with adherence. What commitment would you make related to managing medications? [Ask] Is there a step you can take today towards your commitment for action? Could you share your answer with a peer?	Given lecture, discussion, practice and feedback; The learner will commit to medication adherence; To the extent that three strategies are named; As evaluated by self, peers and therapist/facilitator.

1 minute	Wrap up	[Ask] Are there any questions? [Do] Thank everyone for coming and participating.	Personal response.

Reference

Jimmy B., & Jose J. (2011). Patient Medication Adherence: Measures in Daily Practice. *Oman Medical Journal.* 26(3): 155–159. doi: 10.5001/omj.2011.38.

Reference for Handout

Jimmy B, Jose J. (2011). Patient Medication Adherence: Measures in Daily Practice. *Oman Medical Journal.* 26(3):155–159. doi: 10.5001/omj.2011.38

1.3 Forming Health Habits and Balance in Occupations

LEARNING POINT

Following basic health routines gives a strong foundation for coping with stress.

LEARNING OBJECTIVE

Given experiment, recipe activity, lecture, discussion, practice and feedback;
The learner will commit to a health habit;
To the extent that all in writing, at least four activities are included in a daily schedule and one strategy for habit formation is identified;
As evaluated by self, peers and therapist/facilitator.

MATERIALS

Whiteboard or flipchart and markers, highlighters

HANDOUTS

* Recipe for daily health
* Strategies for forming habits
* My plan to form a health habit

Table 1.3 Forming health habits and balance in occupations

Time frame	Learning stage	Facilitator	Expected learner response
3 minutes	Orientation	[Say] Welcome, etc. [Say] Stress can be defined as how our body adapts to change. The more change we experience, the higher our stress. Basic health habits and consistent routines reduce change, and keep our body and mind prepared for managing stress.	
2 minutes	Clarification	[Say] The objective is: To commit to health habits. [Say] Today we will: • Do a brief experiment • Develop a recipe for health • Discuss benefits and drawbacks of a routine • Review strategies for forming habits • Map out a one-day personal basic routine [Ask] Are we good to go?	Yes.
5 minutes	Warm-up	[Say] Let's try a simple experiment. I would like you to cross your arms. Now cross your arms the opposite way from what you normally do. Hold it that way for a few moments.	Learners participate in experiment.

(continued)

Table 1.3 Cont.

Time frame	Learning stage	Facilitator	Expected learner response
		[Ask] What did crossing your arms in a different way from what you normally do, feel like in terms of comfort, ease and mental effort?	Felt odd, difficult, more concentration needed etc.
		Did it seem less awkward when you held them in that position for a period of time?	Likely yes.
		[Say] Making change can initially be difficult, but with time it can become more comfortable and habitual.	
10 minutes	Experience	[Do] Provide handout: **Recipe for daily health.**	
		[Say] Using the handout, work with a partner to develop a recipe for basic health. Make a recipe that includes six to eight daily occupations that promote health. In your recipe, include a quantity. The handout has an occupation example – eight hours sleep. Share your recipe with the group.	Learners work together to add at least six items to the recipe and present to others.
5 minutes	Reflection	[Ask] How do your recipe items compare to what was captured by others?	Many similarities.
		[Ask] Which activities do you do regularly?	Personal response.

15 minutes	Generalization	[Say] In pairs, identify a health occupation that presents a challenge right now and explain two reasons why. Then discuss two advantages of including that occupation as part of a daily routine. [Say] According to a study by Lally (2010), it takes 18 to 254 days to form a habit with the average being 66 days; it may take 21 days for a simple behaviour change – like having a glass of water at dinner. [Do] Provide handout: **Strategies for forming habits.** Review as a group. [Ask] What strategies would help you form a health habit and why?	Learners participate in discussion. Practice helps learning, tell others for accountability etc.
10 minutes	Application	[Do] Provide handout: **My plan to form a health habit.** [Say] Choose one behaviour change you would like to make in forming a daily health habit. Include your strategies for making the habit stick.	Learners complete the work individually.

(continued)

Table 1.3 Cont.

Time frame	Learning stage	Facilitator	Expected learner response
8 minutes	Evaluation	[Say] Map out a schedule to include at least four activities for basic health. Place a star beside the behaviour change that is a priority for forming a health habit.	Given experiment, recipe activity, lecture, discussion, practice and feedback; The learner will commit to a health habits; To the extent that all in writing, at least four activities are included in a daily schedule and one strategy for habit formation is identified; As evaluated by self, peers and therapist/facilitator.
2 minutes	Wrap up	[Ask] Are there any questions? [Do] Thank everyone for coming and participating.	Personal response.

Reference

Lally, P., van Jaarsveld, C., Potts, H., Wardle, J. (2010). How are habits formed: Modelling habit formation in the real world. *European Journal of Social Psychology. 40(6). 998–1009.* https://doi.org/10.1002/ejsp.674.

Reference for Handouts

Lally, P., van Jaarsveld, C., Potts, H., Wardle, J. (2010). How are habits formed: Modelling habit formation in the real world. *European Journal of Social Psychology. 40(6). 998–1009.* https://doi.org/10.1002/ejsp.674.

1.4 Meal Simplification to Fuel Occupation Engagement

LEARNING POINT

Meal preparation can be simplified to ensure regular meals as a way to care for ourselves.

LEARNING OBJECTIVE

Given recipes ideas, lecture, discussion, practice and feedback;

The learner will construct a one-day menu;

To the extent that in writing, each breakfast, lunch and dinner meals are identified, three strategies to simplify meal preparation are present and one solution to an obstacle is named;

As evaluated by self, peers and therapist/facilitator.

MATERIALS

Whiteboard or flipchart and markers

HANDOUTS

*   Strategies to simplify meal preparation
*   Obstacles and solutions for meal preparation
*   One-day menu

Table 1.4 Meal simplification to fuel occupation engagement

Time frame	Learning stage	Facilitator	Expected learner response
3 minutes	Orientation	[Say] Welcome, etc. [Say] Eating regular, nutritious meals fuels us for occupation. Preparing meals can be time consuming and can sometimes feel overwhelming. Strategies to simplify meal preparation can ease the effort.	
1 minute	Clarification	[Say] The objective is: To construct a menu plan [Say] Today our agenda will include: • Sharing a favourite, simple recipe • Reading strategies to simplify meal preparation • Brainstorming obstacles/solutions for meals • Making a one-day menu and grocery list	
6 minutes	Warm-up	[Say] Share a simple recipe that you make for breakfast, lunch or dinner. Say why it is simple to prepare.	Personal response.
6 minutes	Experience	[Do] Distribute handout: **Strategies to simplify meal preparation**. Invite learners to take turns reading the different strategies on the handout.	Learners take turns reading the handout.

5 minutes	Reflection	[Ask] Have you ever used some of the strategies that are listed on the handout? [Ask] Is there a strategy that seems interesting for you?	Yes/no. Personal response.
22 minutes	Generalization	[Say] In pairs, list three to five obstacles that you face with the preparation of meals and state why. Then name solutions to the obstacles. [Do] Distribute handout: **Obstacles and solutions for meal preparation.** [Say] Here are more examples of obstacles and solutions. Choose one idea to add to your solutions and state how it would further help with meal preparation.	Learners work in pairs to generate lists. Learners complete the activity in pairs.
7 minutes	Application	[Do] Distribute handout: **One-day menu.** [Say] Complete the first part of the handout. In the space provided, write down the top obstacle you are most likely to face with regards to meal preparation. Identify solutions that you can add to your routine to address that obstacle. You can write a barrier that is not listed on the handout.	Learners complete the handout individually.

(continued)

Table 1.3 Cont.

Time frame	Learning stage	Facilitator	Expected learner response
8 minutes	Evaluation	[Say] Complete a one-day menu with recipes for breakfast, lunch and dinner. Include strategies that you will use to simplify the meal preparation. Share two meal strategies with a peer.	Given recipes ideas, lecture, discussion, practice and feedback; The learner will construct a one-day menu; To the extent that in writing, each breakfast, lunch and dinner meals are identified, three strategies to simplify meal preparation are present and one solution to an obstacle is named; As evaluated by self, peers and therapist/facilitator.
2 minutes	Wrap up	[Ask] Are there any questions? [Do] Thank everyone for coming and participating.	Personal response.

References for Handouts

Korb-Khalsa, K., & Leutenberg, E. (1996). *Life Management Skills IV: Reproducible activity handouts created for facilitators.* Beachwood, OH: Wellness Reproductions & Publishing Inc.

Other Resource

Health Canada. (2006). Healthy eating. Retrieved from www.canada.ca/en/health-canada/services/food-nutrition/canada-food-guide/using-food-guide/fast-easy-meal-ideas.html.

1   Handouts

Health and Wellness Routines

1.1 Sleep Hygiene to Improve Daily Occupations

Sleep hygiene checklist

Consider the following tips for better sleep (Peach, Gaultney & Gray, 2016; Mass & Robbins, 2012). Place a checkmark in the column that represents your use of these suggestions.

DAILY SCHEDULE	*Rarely*	*Sometimes*	*Regularly*
Go to sleep at the same time daily, including weekends			
Wake/get up at the same time daily, including weekends			
Follow your medication schedule			
Turn off screens two hours before bed			
Exercise three to six hours before bed			
Drink only caffeine-free beverages 8 hours before bed			
Remain physically, socially and intellectually active			
Use machine for sleep apnea if prescribed			
Eat regular, nutritious meals			
Eat only a light snack if hungry before bed			
Aim for six to ten hours of sleep regularly			
Contact medical doctor if low energy or poor sleep			
Limit alcohol and nicotine intake			
Avoid alcohol three to four hours before bed			

DAILY SCHEDULE (continued)	*Rarely*	*Sometimes*	*Regularly*
Minimize napping (seven hours before sleep time, keep naps to less than one hour)			
Get up after 20 minutes if not sleeping			
Spend time in natural light every day			
Limit time in bed when not sleeping			
SLEEP ENVIRONMENT			
Keep bed free from office/schoolwork and TV			
Keep room cool			
Block bright light (e.g. dark blinds, eye mask, turn clock away from you)			
Limit noise			
Limit sharing bed with kids/pets			
Keep bedroom for sleep and sex only			
RELAXATION			
Listen to quiet music			
Read a dull book before bed			
Focus on pleasant mental images			
Use relaxation techniques, deep breathing			
Have a warm bath more than 2 hours before bed			
MANAGE THOUGHTS			
Set aside worry time earlier in the day			
Review pleasant thoughts or gratitude			
Repeat a calming word as you breathe out (e.g. "one")			
Be realistic in sleep expectations			

References

Mass, J., & Robbins, R. (2012). *Sleep for success! Everything you must know about sleep but are too tired to ask.* Authorhouse: Indiana.

Peach, H., Gaultney, J., & Gray, D. (2016). Sleep hygiene and sleep quality as predictors of positive and negative dimensions of mental health in college students. *Cogent Psychology.* 3(1). https://doi.org/10.1080/23311908.2016.1168768.

Sleep facts

- Adults typically need 7 to 10 hours of sleep, while infants and children may need between 10 to 16 hours per day.
- Late night screen time can impact physical and thought functions (Garett, Liu & Young, 2016).
- Sleep plays an important role in physical, cognitive and emotion function (Fung, Wiseman-Hakes, Stergiou-Kita, Nguyen & Colantonio, 2013).
- Exercise can reduce pain, relax muscles, and improve mood, which can improve restful sleep. Exercise 4 to 6 hours before sleep to allow the body temperature to drop for sleep (Maas, 2012).
- Alcohol before sleep may cause you to feel drowsy, but it interferes with sleep quality that is needed for restoration (Maas, 2012).
- Cannabis reduces sleep quality (Jacobus, Bava, Cohen-Zion, Mahmood & Tapert, 2009).

References

Fung, C., Wiseman-Hakes, C., Stergiou-Kita, M., Nguyen, M., & Colantonio, A. (2013). Time to wake up: Bridging the gap between theory and practice for sleep in occupational therapy. *British Journal of Occupational Therapy.* 76(8) 384–386. https://doi.org/ 10.4276%2F030802213X13757040168432.

Garett, R., Liu, S., & Young, S. (2016). The relationship between social media use and sleep quality among undergraduate students. *Information, Communication & Society.* 21(2) 163–173. https://doi.org/10.1080/1369118X.2016.1266374.

Jacobus, J., Bava, S., Cohen-Zion, M., Mahmood, O., & Tapert, S. (2009). Functional consequences of marijuana use in adolescents. *Pharmacology Biochemistry Behaviour.* 92(4) 559–565. doi: 10.1016/j.pbb.2009.04.001.

Mass, J., & Robbins, R. (2012). *Sleep for success! Everything you must know about sleep but are too tired to ask.* Authorhouse: Indiana.

Card game: Answer sheet

Healthy	*Unhealthy*
Keep bedroom cool to sleep.	Go to bed at different times during the week and on weekends to accommodate a social life.
Get up at the same time during the week and on weekends.	Drink alcohol within three hours of bedtime.
Avoid caffeine (coffee, tea, cola, chocolate) 6 hours before bed.	Share the bed with pets or kids.
Exercise regularly and stop at least 3 hours before bedtime.	Argue with my partner in bed.
Get out of bed after 30 minutes when having difficulty falling or staying asleep and do a quiet activity.	Watch the news or spend time on other screens before turning out the lights.
Stop or reduce smoking.	Do paperwork in bed to wrap it up before going to sleep.
Rotate and flip mattress every 3 months.	Avoid using sleep aid such as a machine for sleep apnea as it bothers my partner.
Learn relaxation techniques such as progressive muscle relaxation, Benson's technique, or autogenic techniques.	Read an exciting book right before sleep time.

My four chosen behaviours to improve sleep quality

Behaviour to improve sleep	Specific action I will take
Example: Reduce caffeine	I will drink water instead of cola. I will switch to herbal teas for a warm drink alternative. If I eat chocolate, it will be at or before my supper hour.
1.	
2.	
3.	
4.	

I am committed to doing behaviour number _____ for the next 48 hours.

One-day schedule

Consider activities/behaviours you can do as part of your daily routine to improve sleep quality such as exercise, a consistent sleep and wake time, designated worry time, relaxation, reducing screen time, and regular meals, etc. Map out a one-day schedule to include those wake-time activities that might improve your sleep time and quality.

Time	Activity

1.2 Medication Adherence as Part of a Healthy Routine

Challenges impacting medication adherence

Medication adherence considers how well a person follows the recommendations of a health care provider. Adherence is boosted when the physician and person consider medical opinion and the person's preferences and lifestyle (Jimmy & Jose, 2011). Medication adherence can impact disease management and reduce relapse. Not taking medications happens for a variety of reasons: Not filling prescriptions; stopping medication; not taking medication as prescribed (Jimmy & Jose, 2011).

Below are examples of reasons why problems arise with medication adherence. Highlight any reasons that have impacted you.

I am afraid about side effects	I do not feel well	I have other demands on my time	The distance to the pharmacy makes it difficult
The instruction for taking medication is too complex	I have negative thoughts such as "it won't help"	I feel well so I think "I don't need it"	Others do not support me taking the medication
I am out during dose time and do not have access	I am not able to renew the prescription	There has been miscommunication with the doctor	I stockpile them for self-harm
I do not like the side effects	I have unanswered questions	I skip doses	I take medication at the wrong time
I feel embarrassment	It seems to take too much effort	I forget	The cost seems too much

Other reasons

Reference

Jimmy B., & Jose J. (2011). Patient Medication Adherence: Measures in Daily Practice. *Oman Medical Journal*. 26(3) 155–159. doi: 10.5001/omj.2011.38.

Possible solutions to improve medication adherence

Check off suggestions below that might help you with medication adherence.

❑ Talk with the doctor about my needs and challenges
❑ Work with the doctor to determine if medication prescription can be simplified (less meds, bi-weekly injection, group together times to take medication)
❑ Use a calendar or schedule to mark off when medications are taken and need renewal
❑ Have pharmacy deliver medication
❑ Use a pill box or blister pack to help remember if medication was taken
❑ Pair taking medication with a habit activity (e.g. put medication by toothbrush or coffee)
❑ Set alarms on phone or other device
❑ Get support from a family member
❑ Carry one dose in your wallet or purse so you can take medication if you are out at dose time
❑ Write down questions for your doctor or pharmacist to ask on next visit
❑ Return expired or unused medication to the pharmacy for disposal
❑ Remind myself of the benefits of taking the medication as prescribed
❑ Talk to a health care professional about possible subsidy programs to offset the cost of medication
❑ Other

1.3 Forming Health Habits and Balance in Occupations

Recipe for daily health

Think of some daily occupations from self-care, productivity or leisure that provide a foundation for basic health. Choose six to eight occupations and these will become the ingredients in your recipe. Do not forget to include the quantity of the ingredient! This recipe has the occupation of sleep as an example.

Quantity	Occupation/Ingredient
Eight hours	Sleep

Strategies for forming habits

It takes 18 to 254 days to form a habit with the average being 66 days (Lally et al., 2010). A common myth is that it only takes 21 days, though this could be true for a simple behaviour change like having a glass of water at dinner. Here are five strategies to increase habit formation (Lally et al., 2010).

Intrinsic motivators: Finding a personal reason to change a habit and it is much more likely to stick over time than rewards or punishments. Consider a minimum quota for the behaviour. For example: *I will walk daily to become stronger,* ***at least once around the block***.

Behaviour chains: Link the new behaviour to something you already do as part of your routine. For example: *I will brush my teeth at night* (regular behaviour) *then take my medication* (new behaviour).

Reduce the options: Narrow your options to keep it simple and to reduce decision-making. For example: *I will eat breakfast every day. I will have cereal, milk, and one piece of fruit.*

Visualize: Instead of visualizing the end result, visualize the process. For example: *Visualize knitting in your favourite chair to improve balance of leisure activity.*

Dodge the "Forget it" trap: The risk when the habit formation becomes a challenge is giving up. Consider where your attempt at change is breaking down and choose a strategy to help. For example: *I want to eat a healthy home-cooked meal instead of take-out for dinner, but I am too tired when I get home from work to decide what to make. I will make a menu plan on the weekend and buy the ingredients I need. That way I do not need to decide what to make after working all day or wonder what food I have available. I just need to prepare the meal and that will be easier.*

Reference

Lally, P., van Jaarsveld, C., Potts, H., & Wardle, J. (2010). How are habits formed: Modelling habit formation in the real world. *European Journal of Social Psychology. 40(6) 998–1009.* https://doi.org/10.1002/ejsp.674.

My plan to form a health habit

A. Name one occupation you are considering to put in your daily routine. Write it in the space below.

B. List two challenges for forming this occupation into a habit.
    1. _____
    2. _____

C. In the space below, list one advantage of doing this occupation regularly?

D. Choose a strategy for forming health habits to make your occupation choice part of your daily routine. Write your strategy in the space below and define how you would use the strategy.

E. Map four health occupations onto a schedule, including the one listed on this sheet.

Time of day	My healthy occupation

1.4 Meal Simplification to Fuel Occupation Engagement

Strategies to simplify meal preparation

Meal preparation can be challenging and takes time. These strategies may simplify meal preparation and speed up the process (Korb-Khalsa & Leutenberg, 1996).

☞ **Use 6 ingredients or less**: By reducing the number of ingredients used, it takes less time to make the recipe. Healthy recipes do not necessarily need lots of ingredients. For example, a simple, healthy meal could be fish cooked with dill and lemon juice, whole grain rice and steamed frozen vegetables.

☞ **Use no more than 2 pots or pans**: When possible, cook everything in the same pan or pot. For example, stir fry chicken and remove from pan, then cook vegetables in the same pan. Return the chicken to the pan with vegetables, add frozen corn and a broth and let simmer until corn is tender. Limit the number of dishes used to reduce clean-up time.

☞ **Choose recipes that require 20 minutes or less to complete**: To reduce preparation time, buy canned or frozen products or cook some food ahead of time.

☞ **Use the slow cooker or instant cooker**: Slow cookers can be started in the morning and cook during the day to be ready in the evening. Instant cookers reduce the cooking time.

☞ **Recruit help**: Dividing meal preparation with someone can speed the process and provide socialization. If cooking with children, assign tasks that match the age of the child.

☞ **Break down the task**: Instead of doing all the food preparation at one time, spread the work over two sessions to conserve your energy. Chopping/cutting can be done in the morning, then assemble the ingredients and cook the meal at night.

Reference

Korb-Khalsa, K., & Leutenberg, E. (1996). *Life Management Skills IV: Reproducible activity handouts created for facilitators.* Beachwood, OH: Wellness Reproductions & Publishing Inc.

Obstacles and solutions for meal preparation

Difficulty deciding what to make:

☞ Plan meals/menu for the upcoming day, week or 2 weeks
☞ Keep some meals similar such as cereal or toast, and a piece of fruit for breakfast every day

Finding nutritious recipes:

☞ Many websites exist with recipes and reviews. Look for categories such as healthy, easy or quick. Some websites allow you to enter ingredients you have on hand for recipe ideas
☞ Build your own cookbook with recipes for breakfast, lunch and dinner
☞ For nutrition tips, the Health Canada website offers free educational resources and recipes www.canada.ca/en/health-canada/services/tips-healthy-eating.html

Fatigue or low energy:

☞ Make a few extra portions when preparing a meal and freeze it for a later day
☞ Keep a few staples in your pantry to put together quick and easy meals
☞ Sit as much as possible when chopping, washing and assembling food
☞ Write your grocery list according to location in the store to cut down on extra steps

Managing costs:

☞ Look at flyers for products on sale. There are apps that have the electronic version of flyers
☞ Buy produce that is in season
☞ Use loyalty programs, points programs and price-match policies of the stores
☞ Reduce food waste by eating leftovers and using what's left of produce in recipes like soup
☞ Make a list of ingredients when shopping to reduce overbuying

Other ideas:

One-day menu

Name an obstacle that you face with meal preparation and identify one solution to address that obstacle.

Obstacle	Solution

A menu plan is one way to simplify the efforts of meal preparation. Complete a one-day menu. Include strategies that you will use to simplify meal preparation.

	Name the recipe or meal idea	Ingredients	Strategies used to reduce time and effort in preparing the meal
Breakfast:			
Lunch:			
Dinner:			

Other resource

Health Canada. (2006). Healthy eating. Retrieved from www.canada.ca/en/health-canada/services/food-nutrition/canada-food-guide/using-food-guide/fast-easy-meal-ideas.html.

2 Modules

Change the Situation

2.1 Overcoming Roadblocks to Change Occupation Performance

LEARNING POINT

There are alternatives when faced with a barrier for making change.

LEARNING OBJECTIVE

Given comparison activity, brainstorm, lecture, discussion, practice and feedback;

The learner will identify one goal towards change;

To the extent that all in writing one barrier for change is identified, two strategies to overcome the barrier are named and the action is defined;

As evaluated by self and therapist/facilitator.

MATERIALS

Whiteboard or flipchart and markers, four symbols for weather posted at various locations around the room (examples could include simple drawings or words to represent: Sunshine; sun with cloud cover; tornado, rainbow.)

DOI: 10.4324/9781003189695-3

HANDOUTS

- Examples of barriers and strategies for making change
- Action plan for change

Table 2.1 Overcoming roadblocks to change occupation performance

Time frame	Learning stage	Facilitator	Expected learner response
2 minutes	Orientation	[Say] Welcome, etc. [Say] There are pros and cons to making changes in our daily lives/routines. Once the decision has been made to make a change, it is helpful to identify possible barriers that may prevent reaching the goal. Naming alternative methods and resources can keep our motivation up as we persist with the change process.	
2 minutes	Clarification	[Say] The objective is: To state one goal towards change. [Say] Today we will: • Do a comparison exercise • Identify possible barriers to making change • Choose solutions to overcome barriers • Write an action plan for making the change [Ask] Are we good to go?	Yes.

(continued)

Table 2.1 Cont.

Time frame	Learning stage	Facilitator	Expected learner response
10 minutes	Warm-up	[Do] Indicate four weather posters around the room. Examples could include: Sunshine, cloud cover, rainbow, tornado.	
		[Say] Think of one change you have been working on recently. Go to the weather poster that best represents how you are progressing with making this change.	
		[Say] Discuss with the other members in your group the reason you chose that weather poster. Then have one representative from your group share the reasons for the choice with the large group.	Learners participate in the task and discussion. Rainbow may represent overcoming struggles, etc.
		[Ask] Did you notice people's choice reflected barriers they are facing or overcoming barriers?	Personal response.
		[Say] Choose a partner and return to a place at the table where you can work together.	Learners pair with others.
10 minutes	Experience	[Do] Provide pairs with a large piece of flipchart paper and markers.	

Time	Section		
		[Say] Divide your paper into two vertical sections. With your partner, brainstorm a list of barriers to successful change on the left section of your paper, and possible solutions to the barriers on the right side.	Barriers: Financial constraints, low energy, fear, not aware of resources, etc. Solutions: Do small steps, follow the plan and not the feeling, positive self-talk, etc.
		[Do] Post the lists around the room.	
		[Say] Take a moment to look at the barriers and solutions identified from other pairs.	Learners review lists.
7 minutes	Reflection	[Ask] Were there any similarities? What differences did you notice?	Yes, and name them.
		[Say] Think of a past successful change you made. Identify a roadblock you encountered from one of the pairs' worksheets. Tell us about the roadblock and a strategy you used to overcome the barrier.	Personal response.
		[Ask] Is there a strategy that you would like to further develop?	Personal response.
5 minutes	Generalization	[Ask] What are the risks of making change?	Risks: Emotions such as guilt, fear, frustration, new responsibilities and pushback from others, etc.

(continued)

Table 2.1 Cont.

Time frame	Learning stage	Facilitator	Expected learner response
		[Ask] What are the benefits of making change?	Benefits: Success, gaining control, new knowledge/skills, etc.
12 minutes	Application	[Say] Here is a scenario. A friend, Liza has asked to meet with you to discuss a change she wants to make. She tends to isolate herself when she is feeling down and this feeds into a greater sense of loneliness and depression. She would like to have more contact with others and be more involved in her community. [Do] Provide handout: **Examples of barriers and strategies for making change.** [Say] In groups of three, use the handout to highlight three strategies that you could coach Liza on to assist with making change. Discuss one reason for each of your choices.	Learners complete discussion in triads.

| 10 minutes | Evaluation | [Do] Provide handout: **Action plan for change.**

[Say] Complete the worksheet for a personal behaviour change you are considering or are working on. List a benefit of making this change. Indicate a roadblock or barrier that you have encountered or are anticipating. List two strategies to overcome this roadblock. Consider if there is a resource you could use to help you with this change.
Write a specific action to work on the change this week.

[Do] Circulate among learners to check progress on work sheet and provide coaching as needed. | Given comparison activity, brainstorm, lecture, discussion, practice and feedback; The learner will identify one goal towards change; To the extent that all in writing one barrier for change is identified, two strategies to overcome the barrier are named and the action is defined; As evaluated by self and therapist/facilitator. |
| 2 minutes | Wrap up | [Ask] Are there any questions?

[Do] Thank everyone for coming and participating. | Personal response. |

2.2 Building Community Networks to Increase Opportunities for Occupation

LEARNING POINT

A sense of belonging is a valuable coping tool that can be strengthened by accessing community resources.

LEARNING OBJECTIVE

Given brainstorm, pamphlets, maps, lecture, electronic resources (optional), discussion, practice and feedback;

The learner will identify one community resource;

To the extent that one organization is named, the address and phone number are listed, hours of operation are identified and one personal interest about the resource is shared with a peer;

As evaluated by self, peers and therapist/facilitator.

MATERIALS

Whiteboard or flipchart and markers, pamphlets/printouts of various local community resources (approximately 10 in total including peer support/support group, professional support such as the crisis line, a volunteer organization, community activities, a walking club, an interest course, church, etc.), and/or access to computer (iPad, cell phone with data).

HANDOUTS

- Expanding my community network

Table 2.2 Building community networks to increase opportunities for occupation

Time frame	Learning stage	Facilitator	Expected learner response:
3 minutes	Orientation	[Say] Welcome, etc. [Say] Developing healthy relationships is an important life skill. Connecting to community resources provides opportunity to make these relationship connections.	
1 minutes	Clarification	[Say] The objective is: To identify a community resource. [Say] Today we will: • Brainstorm different community resources • Discuss barriers of accessing these resources • Identify strategies to overcome the barriers • Locate a community resource of personal interest [Ask]: Are we good to go?	Yes.
3 minutes	Warm-up	[Say] Let's brainstorm different ways to find out about community resources.	Local newspaper, meet up apps, word of mouth, church, brochures, community centre, library, computer search, etc.
10 minutes	Experience	[Do] Provide brochures or printouts on local community resources.	

(continued)

Table 2.2 Cont.

Time frame	Learning stage	Facilitator	Expected learner response:
		[Say] Take a look at each of the brochures and pass them around.	Learners scan the material.
10 minutes	Reflection	[Ask] Did you recognize a resource that you have heard of or used?	Yes/No
		[Ask] Did any resources capture your interest in some way?	Personal response
		[Say] Please identify a community resource you have used in the past and tell us how it was helpful to you.	Personal response
12 minutes	Generalization	[Say] In pairs, choose two barriers that might keep you from accessing community resources. Then identify one or two strategies for each that could help tackle the barrier. When finished, share your ideas with the large group.	Finances – look for free items, Knowledge – ask others, Emotions –explore a resource through small steps (find the location, call administration), Wait lists – ask to be put on a cancellation list
10 minutes	Application	[Do] Provide handout: **Expanding my community network.**	

		[Say] Choose two ideas for expanding your community network from the following 5 categories. For each idea, name three action steps you can take to progress toward using this community network.	Personal response (Example: Community activity – I will contact the community centre to ask about free activities in our neighbourhood, I will find out the times and locations, I will name one positive reason for joining.
10 minutes	Evaluation	[Say] Next, refer to the "My community resource" section of the same handout. Determine one community resource you can use to help build your network. Name the resource and find the address and a contact number. Name the hours of operation. [Say] Share one reason for your interest in this resource with a peer.	Given brainstorm, pamphlets, maps, lecture, electronic resources (optional), discussion, practice and feedback; The learner will identify one community resource; To the extent that one organization is named, the address and phone number are listed, hours of operation are identified and one personal interest about the resource is shared with a peer; As evaluated by self, peers and therapist/facilitator.
1 minute	Wrap up	[Ask] Are there any questions? [Do] Thank everyone for coming and participating.	Personal response.

2.3 Defining Healthy Boundaries

LEARNING POINT

Defining boundaries in relationships can offer predictability and safety.

LEARNING OBJECTIVE

Given boundary demonstration, lecture, discussion, practice and feedback;

The learner will define a healthy boundary;

To the extent that one personal boundary violation is named and a constructive change is described;

As evaluated by self, peers and therapist/facilitator.

MATERIALS

Whiteboard or flipchart and markers

HANDOUTS

- Boundaries versus walls
- Defining boundaries
- Personal scenario

Table 2.3 Defining healthy boundaries

Time frame	Learning stage	Facilitator	Expected learner response
3 minutes	Orientation	[Say] Welcome, etc. [Say] Boundaries are an important consideration for healthy relationships. They define personal values, protect us, and allow us to make good choices for living, giving, loving and relating (Black & Enns, 1998). Boundaries promote self-care and self-respect. The first step is to recognize the nature of healthy boundaries.	
2 minutes	Clarification	[Say] The objective is: To define healthy boundaries. [Say] Today we will: • Participate in a boundary demonstration • Define characteristics of boundaries • Explore boundaries to increase health [Ask] Are we good to go?	Yes.
5 minutes	Warm-up	[Ask] What are some behaviour expectations within this group today? [Do] Capture ideas on whiteboard or flip chart.	Take turns, keep information confidential, limit interruptions, come on time, finish on time, keep self and others safe, communicate in a calm manner.

(continued)

Table 2.3 Cont.

Time frame	Learning stage	Facilitator	Expected learner response
		[Ask] What is the purpose of defining these expectations?	To set expectations of acceptable behaviour, etc.
5 minutes	Experience	[Do] Divide group into pairs.	Learners participate in demonstration.
		[Say] In pairs, stand 20 steps away from your partner. One person will slowly approach the partner. The person standing still is to say, "stop" at the closest point of comfort. This would be the edge of a personal space boundary. Note the distance between each other and other pairs. Then you and your partner will reverse roles.	
6 minutes	Reflection	[Ask] Was the distance the same or different between trials?	Yes/no
		What was your comfort level in saying, "stop"?	Personal response
		Was the person approaching you surprised with the distance between you and your partner when asked to stop?	Yes/no
		What about the distances observed in other pairs?	Likely surprised at differences between groups

11 minutes	Generalization	[Say] There are many different areas of our lives in which we define our boundaries including: Physical (closeness to others, personal property, decisions about our body); Emotional (love needs, privacy, autonomy for choices, responsibilities to others); Social (types of friendships, respect, assistance offered by others); and Mental (ideas we subject ourselves to, learning needs, our right to our own beliefs) (Katherine, 2000).	
		[Ask] What might be factors that could influence the level of comfort with space between self and others?	Gender, familiarity, crowded situations, size, smiling, individual preference, etc.
		[Ask] What does this mean: "Good fences make good neighbours"?	Clear boundaries reduce conflict by setting clear expectations.
		[Do] Provide handout: **Boundaries versus walls.**	
		[Say] In pairs, identify differences between a boundary and a wall, and write them on your handout. Share answers with the large group.	Boundaries: Flexible, discriminate, let safe people in, keep unsafe people out. Walls: Imprison, keep everyone out, instill fear of new experiences.

(continued)

Table 2.3 Cont.

Time frame	Learning stage	Facilitator	Expected learner response
		[Ask] What do healthy boundaries do for you?	Bring order, define your identity, attract respectful relationships.
17 minutes	Application	[Say] In pairs, come up with another metaphor for a boundary. Referring to your metaphor, explain further ideas of what a boundary can do for you.	Cell wall – keeps good nutrients in, throws out toxins. Keys to car – you decide who drives it and rides in it. Border guard – keeps out harm, friendly but choosy.
		[Do] Provide handout: **Defining boundaries** and review. [Say] This summary sheet touches on many of the points we have discussed so far today. Add your ideas to this handout.	Learners add ideas individually.

10 minutes	Evaluation	[Do] Provide handout: **Personal scenario.** [Say] Identify a personal scenario where you would like to define healthier boundaries. Next, explain the nature of the boundary violation; in other words, how does it affect your self-care and self-respect? Write it out on your worksheet. Finally, define a healthier boundary for your personal scenario. Describe the differences or changes you would like to see.	Given boundary demonstration, lecture, discussion, practice and feedback; The learner will define a healthy boundary; To the extent that one personal boundary violation is named and a constructive change is described; As evaluated by self, peers and therapist/facilitator.
1 minute	Wrap up	[Ask] Are there any questions? [Do] Thank everyone for coming and participating.	Personal response.

References

Black, J., & Enns, G. (1998). *Better boundaries: Owning and treasuring your life.* Oakland, CA: New Harbinger Publications.

Katherine, A. (2000). *Where to draw the line: How to set healthy boundaries everyday.* New York, NY: Touchstone.

References for Handouts

Black, J., & Enns, G.,(1998). *Better boundaries: Owning and treasuring your life.* Oakland, CA: New Harbinger Publications.

Katherine, A. (2000). *Where to draw the line: How to set healthy boundaries everyday.* New York, NY: Touchstone.

2.4 Setting Healthy Boundaries to Support Meaningful Occupation

LEARNING POINT

Statements for healthy boundaries.

LEARNING OBJECTIVE

Given game, scenarios, lecture, role play, discussion, practice and feedback;

The learner will construct a statement for a personal boundary;

To the extent that one type of violation is identified, one rule is named, one sentence stem is chosen, a limit is set, and then the statement is role played with a partner;

As evaluated by self, peers and therapist/facilitator.

MATERIALS

Whiteboard or flipchart and markers, paper, pencil, basket

HANDOUTS

- Is this a boundary violation?
- Tips for setting boundaries
- Personal rules for boundaries

Table 2.4 Setting healthy boundaries to support meaningful occupation

Time frame	Learning stage	Facilitator	Expected learner response
3 minutes	Orientation	[Say] Welcome, etc. [Say] A boundary is a limit between you and others. Boundaries define what you will do or not do and what behaviours you will or will not welcome from others. Boundaries define where your feelings, opinions and responsibilities lie and the ownership of others' feelings, opinions and responsibilities (Katherine, 2000). It is an important coping strategy to know how to set boundaries with others – especially those who are exhibiting controlling, critical, manipulative or aggressive behaviours.	
2 minutes	Clarification	[Say] The objective is: To construct a statement for a personal boundary [Say] Today we will: • Participate in a game related to setting limits • Look at scenarios and decide if they are boundary violations • Review risks and benefits of setting boundaries • Choose sentence starters for setting limits • Develop rules for personal boundaries	

(continued)

Table 2.4 Cont.

Time frame	Learning stage	Facilitator	Expected learner response
8 minutes	Warm-up	[Ask] Are we good to go?	Yes.
		[Say] Imagine you are eating some delicious finger food. An acquaintance comes by and grabs some off your plate without asking. Write down what you would say/do, fold your response and place it in this basket.	Learners write individual answers.
		[Say] I will read out all the responses. The first person to my right will repeat one statement and guess who said it. If correct, that person can guess again. If incorrect, the person that was wrongly guessed will have a turn. We will continue until all the answers have been connected to the correct writer.	Learners participate in the game.
		[Say] The answers are unique because we all may have different boundaries or we may have difficulty setting limits.	
5 minutes	Experience	[Do] Provide handout: **Is this a boundary violation?**	Learners take turns reading the statements and answer yes or no if a boundary violation exists.
		[Say] Let's read the following statements and decide if a boundary violation exists.	

5 minutes	Reflection	[Say] Boundary violations can impact time, privacy, possessions, relationships, and physical, mental, emotional or social comfort. [Ask] What would be examples of boundary violations from the handout?	Emotional: Cancelling plans; Social: Friend's relationship; Time: Sister is late; Privacy: Details of illness; Possessions: Taking the car.
15 minutes	Generalization	[Ask] What makes it difficult to set healthy boundaries sometimes? Explain. [Ask] What are the benefits? Explain. [Do] Provide handout: **Tips for setting boundaries** and review out loud the suggested words and phrases for setting boundaries. [Ask] What would be the challenge of using these words or phrases? Explain why.	Fear of anger or rejection, a sense of obligation, dependency for another need fulfillment (such as we rely on them for our ride home) You learn to listen and trust yourself; You take better care of yourself, etc. Emotional discomfort; Not practiced in using these statements, etc.

(continued)

Table 2.4 Cont.

Time frame	Learning stage	Facilitator	Expected learner response
8 minutes	Application	[Ask] What could be words of self-encouragement to assist you in setting a boundary? [Say] Return to the examples of boundary violations we looked at in the beginning of the group (from handout: **Is this a boundary violation?**). Work with a partner. Choose one boundary violation example each and one phrase to respond to the example.	Example: If fear of anger, remind self that you can't make everyone happy all the time; Fear of rejection – not setting limits is no guarantee that I will not be rejected. Personal response.
12 minutes	Evaluation	[Do] Provide handout: **Personal rules for boundaries**. [Say] Let's read through this handout with examples. Next identify one personal boundary violation you are experiencing. Construct a personal rule related to the boundary and develop a statement reflecting application of this rule. Share this information with a partner.	Given game, scenarios, lecture, role play, discussion, practice and feedback; The learner will construct a statement for a personal boundary; To the extent that one type of violation is identified, one rule is named, one sentence stem is chosen, a limit is set,

		and then the statement is role played with a partner; As evaluated by self, peers and therapist/facilitator.	Personal response.
2 minutes	Wrap up	[Ask] Are there any questions? [Do] Thank everyone for coming and participating.	

Reference

Katherine, A. (2000). *Where to draw the line: How to set healthy boundaries everyday.* New York, NY: Touchstone.

References for handouts

Katherine, A. (2000). *Where to draw the line: How to set healthy boundaries everyday.* New York, NY: Touchstone.

Korb-Khalsa, K., & Leutenberg, E. (1999). *Life management skills V: Reproducible activity handouts created for facilitators.* Beachwood, OH: Wellness Reproductions and Publishing Inc.

2   Handouts
Change the Situation

2.1 Overcoming Roadblocks to Change Occupation Performance

Examples of barriers and strategies for making change

Fear of failure: Fear of failure or setbacks can reflect a lack of trust in oneself.

Strategies:

- Remind self that setbacks are a normal part of change, are temporary and provide opportunities to learn what is working and not working
- Say "I will not worry what others think, I will follow my goals and values"
- Follow the plan and not the emotions
- Remember that even if not completely successful, there are gains to be made in trying
- Gather information about the area of change to improve confidence
- Learn relaxation strategies
- Give self credit for small successes

Low motivation: Sometimes the effort of change seems magnified by dwelling on past mistakes, perceived limitations or other obligations. Continuing with the way things are may seem easier and therefore more acceptable than making the change.

Strategies:

- Create a pros and cons list of making the change to determine if the benefits out-weigh the costs. Even difficult changes can be made if we have buy-in that it is truly to our benefit
- Ask self questions such as "How badly do I want it?" "Could I continue even if I feel anxiety?"
- Set aside time to work on tasks when energy and motivation are highest
- Schedule in rewards for completion of small steps of task
- Follow the five-minute rule: work on the task for 5 minutes and then if you want to continue you can. If you want to stop, you still get full credit for working on the task that day. Often once the task is started, it is easier to continue on it

Examples of barriers and strategies for making change (continued)

Distressing emotions (guilt, embarrassment, frustration): Emotions can be triggered by negative self-talk, needing to set limits with others, or asking others for help.

Strategies:

- Remind self that making change may mean giving something else up and saying "no" to something else eventually
- Learn assertiveness skills to communicate your feelings and needs to others
- Learn to recognize negative thoughts and techniques to reframe the thoughts
- Keep in regular contact with supports so that asking for help becomes more comfortable
- Practice mindfulness techniques
- Remind self that I deserve and am responsible for my health, before I look after others

Lack of preparation and resources: First steps may focus on preparing a plan, making decisions and mapping out timelines before action of the actual change begins. Consider resources such as time, energy, knowledge, skill level and finances needed to complete the task.

Strategies:

- Map a timeline and say the steps and stages involved in making the change
- Use an agenda to set aside regular time to work on the goal in small steps
- Limit distractions such as TV, computer, phone to improve concentration
- Consider if any part of the task could be delegated
- Consider asking a community resource or friend to assist you
- Have patience

What three strategies would you coach Liza (from case study example) on to assist with her goal to have more contact with others and be more involved in her community? Discuss one reason for each choice.

Action plan for change

Describe one behaviour change you are considering in the space below.

List a benefit for you to make this change.

What is one roadblock you have encountered or anticipate in making this change?

List two strategies to manage this roadblock. Consider if there is a resource you can use to help you with this change.

1.

2.

What is one specific action step you can take today to work towards this change?

2.2 Building Community Networks to Increase Opportunities for Occupation

Expanding my community network

Choose **two** ideas for expanding your community network from the following five categories. For each of your two ideas, name three action steps you can take to progress towards using this community resource.

   As part of your action steps, you might consider research, discussing with others, or making a visit, etc.

Support group:
   I will locate and join a support group. I will take the following action steps.

- _____

Community activity/event:
   I will attend the following community activity on a regular basis. I will take the following action steps.

- _____

Special interest activity or course:
   I will join a class or scheduled activity. I will take the following action steps.

- _____

Volunteer work:
   I will volunteer. I will take the following action steps.

- _____

Other:
   I will expand my social network by _____
   I will take the following action steps.

- _____

   I will expand my social network by _____
   I will take the following action steps.

- _____

Expanding my community network (continued)

My community resource

Name:

Address:

Phone number:

Hours of operation:

My next step:

2.3 Defining Healthy Boundaries

Boundaries versus walls

Consider the adage "good fences make good neighbours." What does this mean? What does it have to do with personal boundaries?

A clear boundary will reduce or eliminate conflicts by setting clear expectations (Katherine, 2000). There is a difference between a boundary and a wall. Identify differences in the spaces below.

BOUNDARIES	WALLS

Consider a metaphor for personal boundaries – boundary and fence.

Example: A boundary is a fence with a gate that surrounds you and you hold the control to open and close the gate. In a similar way, you are the control centre for your life. You are able to choose and decide what is good for you, what or who is allowed to enter. You also get to decide what is not in your best interest and keep that out.

Come up with another metaphor for personal boundaries. Describe it in the space below.

(*Alternative option: Name two benefits of personal boundaries*)

Reference

Katherine, A. (2000). *Where to draw the line: How to set healthy boundaries everyday.* New York, NY: Touchstone.

Defining boundaries

A personal boundary is a line you draw to protect all or part of your life from the people, thoughts, actions, and behaviours that are not in your best interest for self-care and self-respect (Katherine, 2000). Your boundaries distinguish your feelings, responsibilities and needs from others.

A boundary is:

- A clear line between what is you and not you
- A clear line between what you will and will not put up with
- A clear line between what you have control over and what you do not

What do boundaries do for you?

- Boundaries define your values, beliefs and preferences
- Boundaries offer protection and safety
- Boundaries reduce chaos and offer predictability
- Boundaries encourage respect in relationships
- Boundaries provide reminders of your goals, purpose and of what is meaningful

(Black & Enns, 1998)

What can boundaries do for you?

Examples: Experience new peace and calm, enjoy those people who enrich you, less time repairing your life and more time enhancing it, gain a sense of control over your life, take intelligent risks because you will know how to set limits to protect yourself, etc.).

Other:

References

Black, J., & Enns, G., (1998). *Better boundaries: Owning and treasuring your life.* Oakland, CA: New Harbinger Publications.

Katherine, A. (2000). *Where to draw the line: How to set healthy boundaries everyday.* New York, NY: Touchstone.

Personal scenario

Identify a personal scenario where you would like to have better boundaries in the space below.

```
┌─────────────────────────────────────────────────────────────┐
│                                                               │
│                                                               │
│                                                               │
│                                                               │
│                                                               │
│                                                               │
│                                                               │
│                                                               │
└─────────────────────────────────────────────────────────────┘
```

Explain the boundary violation in the scenario you described? In other words, how is it impacting your self-care? How is it impacting your self-respect? Write your ideas in the space below.

```
┌─────────────────────────────────────────────────────────────┐
│                                                               │
│                                                               │
│                                                               │
│                                                               │
│                                                               │
│                                                               │
└─────────────────────────────────────────────────────────────┘
```

How would you define a healthier boundary in your personal scenario? Describe what differences or changes you would like to see in the space below.

```
┌─────────────────────────────────────────────────────────────┐
│                                                               │
│                                                               │
│                                                               │
│                                                               │
│                                                               │
│                                                               │
│                                                               │
└─────────────────────────────────────────────────────────────┘
```

2.4 Setting Healthy Boundaries to Support Meaningful Occupation

Is this a boundary violation?

1. An acquaintance asks you about the details of your illness that you consider are too personal.
2. A neighbour wants to share intimate details about her life that you would rather not hear.
3. A colleague at work, with whom you share a computer, opens your e-mail marked "personal."
4. Your mother ignores you when you are speaking to her.
5. You agree to meet your sister for lunch at a specific time and she arrives 20 minutes late.
6. Last week your brother asked to borrow your car and you agreed. Today you come home to find he has borrowed it again without permission.
7. You and your partner have made plans for the weekend that you are really looking forward to. When you get home, he tells you he has made other plans without asking you.
8. Your best friend has had an argument with her partner, so you visit the partner to try to patch things up between them.
9. A co-patient in hospital is having a really hard night, so you stay up and sit with her even though you are really tired and it makes you upset too.
10. Your roommate continues to play loud music while you are trying to study, even after you have asked for it to be turned down.

Provide examples from the scenarios for the following boundary violations:

Emotional

Social

Time

Privacy

Possessions

Tips for setting boundaries

Reminders:

- Be clear and to the point without aggression
- Be prepared to feel anxiety, fear, shame or guilt
- Remember that you cannot always take care of someone else's feelings
- Identify symptoms and behaviours that indicate a need for boundaries to be set (anger, resentment, gossip, complaining)
- Remind yourself of benefits of setting boundaries (e.g. getting a sense of control back, teaching others how you would like to be treated)
- Remember that others will have boundaries as well and may not agree with yours
- Follow through on the boundary that is set

Words/phrases for communicating personal boundaries to others (Korb-Khalsa & Leutenberg, 1999)

• I am not interested in …	• This is not in my best interest
• This is not my responsibility	• I do not want to do this
• Yes, I do mind	• I have a problem with …
• That is not acceptable	• I hear what you are saying but …
• That is inappropriate	• I am not comfortable with …
• This is what I need	• We will have to agree to disagree
• I think we see things differently	• Other:

Choose two or three phrases you might consider using to communicate a personal boundary and highlight them in some way.

Reference

Korb-Khalsa, K., & Leutenberg, E. (1999). *Life management skills V: Reproducible activity handouts created for facilitators.* Beachwood, OH: Wellness Reproductions and Publishing Inc.

Personal rules for boundaries

There are many different areas of our lives in which we define our boundaries including:

- Physical: Closeness to others, personal property, decisions about our body
- Emotional: Love needs, privacy, autonomy for choices, responsibilities to others
- Social: Types of friendships, respect, assistance offered by others
- Mental: Ideas we subject ourselves to, learning needs, our right to our own beliefs (Katherine, 2000)

Personal boundaries are defined by rules. Similar to "house rules," these rules define where we will draw the line about what we are willing to tolerate and what we will not tolerate. See the example that follows:

a. What boundary violation are you experiencing? *Watching violent movies interferes with my sleep.*
b. Personal rule: *I will not watch movies with graphic violence.*
c. Application of rule: *I will review the movie content before agreeing to see a movie.*

Further examples of boundary violations, personal rule and statement of application:

1. Pollution: I do not allow smoking in my house. Smokers will be asked to smoke outside.
2. Responsibility: I am not responsible for the financial security of my extended family. I will set limits on loaning them money.
3. Gossip: I will not participate in gossip. If gossip occurs, I will suggest we change the subject.

Write a personal example of a boundary violation:

What is the boundary violation you are experiencing? (Examples: Time, emotions, privacy, possessions, physical, etc.)

What is your personal rule related to this boundary?

How will you apply the personal rule in a situation?

What word or phrase could you use to communicate your personal boundary to others?

Sometimes we may feel fear, guilt or worry about rejection when setting a boundary. What could be words of self-encouragement to assist you in setting this boundary?

Reference

Katherine, A. (2000). *Where to draw the line: How to set healthy boundaries everyday.* New York, NY: Touchstone.

3 Modules

Change Body Response to Stress

3.1 Behaviour Activation to Assist With Initiating Occupation

LEARNING POINT

Activation methods include movement, pleasure and mastery as well as a motivational approach, which emphasizes personal control and choice.

LEARNING OBJECTIVE

Given experiments, lecture, superhero symbol, discussion, practice and feedback;
The learner will explain a behaviour activation strategy;
To the extent that one personal problem activity is named, one strategy from six options is chosen and a plan to use it in the next 24 hours is defined;
As evaluated by self, peers and therapist/facilitator.

MATERIALS

Whiteboard or flipchart and markers, scrap paper, pens, basket for game

DOI: 10.4324/9781003189695-4

HANDOUTS

- Behaviour experiment
- Getting unstuck
- Overcoming avoidance
- Action initiative

Table 3.1 Behaviour Activation to Assist with Initiating Occupation

Time frame	Learning stage	Facilitator	Expected learner response
3 minutes	Orientation	[Say] Welcome, etc. [Say] Sometimes the stress we experience causes us to freeze or avoid action. "Not doing" leads to further avoidance, creating a vicious cycle of inactivity or "why try" type of thinking. Behaviour activation strategies engage the person at the physical, emotional and cognitive levels to move towards action, pleasure and achievement (Greenberger & Padesky, 2016).	
2 minutes	Clarification	[Say] The objective is: To explain behaviour activation strategies. [Say] Today we will: • Carry out some experiments • Determine strategies to improve activation • Write a plan for use of strategies	

(continued)

Table 3.1 Cont.

Time frame	Learning stage	Facilitator	Expected learner response
		[Ask] Are we good to go?	Yes.
10 minutes	Warm-up	[Say] Think of one thing you did to help you get out of bed and start your day today. Ensure it is something you are willing to share with others. Write it on a piece of paper and place it in the basket.	
		[Say] This is a guessing game. I will read the answers out loud and the first person will have a chance to guess who said what. If your answer is guessed correctly, then you get the next guess. If the guess is incorrect, the turn goes to the next person.	Learners participate in the game. Personal responses might include listening to music, having a shower, etc.
		Alternative if less than four people: [Say] Think of one thing you did to help you get out of bed to start your day today. Ensure it is something you are willing to share with others. Choose a symbol or word to represent this idea and put it on a piece of paper. Share your work with the large group.	

		[Say] What you identified is a strategy to assist you to become activated after waking up. We will come back to these strategies later and group them into specific categories.	
8 minutes	Experience	[Do] Provide handout: **Behaviour experiment**.	Learners complete the exercise individually.
		[Say] Please rate your mood in the pre-test section of the handout, on a scale of 1 to 10. 1 = the worst, 10 = the best.	
		[Say] Please do each of the following tasks: • Share something positive that you completed or did in the past • Move your arms up above your head and down again five times • In sitting, lift each knee for five repetitions • Identify one thing you like in the room. Share with the group • Smile or laugh (even if you have to force it)	Learners comply to each request, one at a time.
		[Say] Return to your handout. Rate your mood on the post-test scale, 1 = the worst, 10 = the best.	Learners complete the exercise individually.
10 minutes	Reflection	[Ask] What happened to your mood rating?	Likely mood improved, it is also possible mood showed no change or went down.

(continued)

Table 3.1 Cont.

Time frame	Learning stage	Facilitator	Expected learner response
		[Ask] Do you feel more energy now after completing the experiments?	Yes or no, but likely yes.
		[Ask] How would you describe the difficulty of the experiment activities?	Most will say easy.
		[Do] Invite everyone to write the three summary words: Movement, pleasure, and mastery, on their handout.	
		[Ask] What word from the three choices of movement, pleasure or mastery would you use to summarize each activity from the experiment?	Something likeable = pleasure Task completion = mastery Arm and leg lifts = movement Smile = pleasure
		[Ask] Do you remember your strategy from the warm-up exercise that helped you get out of bed today? Did it relate to movement, pleasure or mastery?	Personal response
12 minutes	Generalization	[Say] Return to the handout: **Behaviour experiment**. In pairs discuss reasons why movement, pleasure or mastery impacts mood and energy.	Learners share their answers with a partner.

Movement gets blood/oxygen pumping to the muscles, feels good.
Pleasure focuses our thoughts on positives. Positive thoughts boost mood while negative thoughts lead to more distress.
Mastery boosts confidence and gives a sense of control.

[Say] Let's have each pair share one idea with the larger group related to why movement, pleasure and mastery impact mood and/or energy.

[Do] Provide handout: **Getting unstuck.**

[Say] From cognitive behaviour theory, behaviour activation methods focus on these three principles of movement, pleasure and mastery (Greenberger & Padesky, 2016). This handout includes reasons why these principles can boost mood. A fourth category for behaviour activation is overcoming avoidance (Greenberger & Padesky, 2016).

[Do] Provide handout: **Overcoming avoidance.**

[Say] Let's review the following ideas for overcoming avoidance (timed/graded tasks, prediction log) by reading through the handout.

(continued)

Table 3.1 Cont.

Time frame	Learning stage	Facilitator	Expected learner response
		[Say] For each category, highlight one point that would be helpful to remember when you are feeling stuck and need to become activated.	Learners participate in highlighting helpful points.
5 minutes	Application	[Say] With a partner, take turns being an Activation Superhero. Choose a symbol or word to represent one effective way to battle your arch-enemy "Sticky Inertia." Your power can be related to one of the activation ideas: Movement, pleasure, mastery, small steps, 5-minute rule or prediction log. Share your symbol with a partner and state one activity that this power allows you to do. For example: A superhero symbol could be *Smiling*, which is related to the power of *Pleasure*. The power of smiling could be used when meeting new people because it relaxes others, and it helps with feeling calm.	Learners participate in activity.

9 minutes	Evaluation	[Do] Provide handout: **Action initiative.** [Say] Write down a task you have difficulty doing in your day or that you have been avoiding. Choose a strategy to help you get unstuck with this task. Define how you will put this strategy into action in the next 24 hours on the worksheet provided. Share with a peer or large group.	Given experiments, lecture, superhero symbol, discussion, practice and feedback; The learner will explain a behaviour activation strategy; To the extent that all in writing one personal problem activity is named, one strategy from six options is chosen and a plan to use it in the next 24 hours is defined; As evaluated by self, peers and therapist/facilitator.
1 minute	Wrap up	[Ask] Are there any questions? [Do] Thank everyone for coming and participating.	Personal response.

Reference

Greenberger, D., & Padesky, C. (2016). *Mind over mood: Change how you feel by changing the way you think:* (2nd ed.). *New York, NY: Guilford Press.*

References for Handouts

Biddle S., & Mutrie, N. (2001). Psychology of physical activity: Determinants, well-being and interventions. *Medicine & Science.* Routledge, London. doi: 10.4324/9780203019320 Source: OAI.

Bourne, E. (2020). *The anxiety and phobia workbook* (7th ed.). Oakland, CA: New Harbinger Publications. Cole, M. B. (2008).

Gabora, I. (2002). Cognitive mechanisms underlying the creative process. In T. Hewett & T. Kavanaugh (Eds.), *Proceedings of the Fourth International Conference on Creativity and Cognition, 13–16 October* (pp. 126–133). Leicestershire, UK: Loughborough University.

Greenberger, D., & Padesky, C. (2016). *Mind over mood: Change how you feel by changing the way you think: (2nd ed.). New York, NY: Guilford Press.*

Hutton, D. (2008). Play. In J. Creek and L. Lougher (Eds.), *Occupational therapy and mental health, fourth edition.* (pp. 345–358). Philadelphia: Churchill Livingstone Elsevier.

Krupa, T., Edgelow, M., Chen, S., Mieras, C., Almas, A., Perry, A., & Bransfield, M. (2010). *Action over inertia: Addressing the activity-health needs of individuals with serious mental illness.* Ottawa, On. CAOT publications ACE.

Perrin, T. (2001). Don't despise the fluffy bunny: A reflection from practice. *The British Journal of Occupational Therapy, 64,* 129–134. doi: 10.1177/030802260106400304.

Royeen, C. (1997). Play as occupation and as an indicator in health. In B. Chandler (Ed.). The essence of play: A child's occupation. American Occupational Therapy Association, Bethesda, Maryland. (pp. 1–14).

US Department of Health and Human Services (1996). Physical activity and health: A report of the Surgeon General (Executive summary). Superintendent of documents. Pittsburgh, PA.

3.2 Anger Management Strategies for Constructive Action

LEARNING POINT

Developing strategies to act versus react to anger is a choice.

LEARNING OBJECTIVE

Given game, lecture, discussion, practice and feedback;
The learner will develop an anger management plan;
To the extent that all in writing, four action steps are identified and two personal responsibilities are named;
As evaluated by self, peers and therapist/facilitator.

MATERIALS

Game template transformed onto white board or flipchart (see game template and resource for therapist/instructor), markers, statements for game outlining symptoms, thoughts and behaviours related to anger emotions, blank paper for each participant.

HANDOUT

- Game template and resource for therapist/facilitator
- Anger game: Answers
- Strategies for changing thoughts, behaviours and physical symptoms of anger
- Anger management plan

Table 3.2 Anger Management Strategies for Constructive Action

Time frame	Learning stage	Facilitator	Expected learner response
3 minutes	Orientation	[Say] Welcome, etc. [Say] Anger is a natural emotion that is important for survival (Greenberger & Padesky, 2016). It can range in intensity from annoyed to enraged. It occurs in response to a perceived threat and can trigger a physical response. Actions related to anger can be constructive or destructive. It is our choice and responsibility which actions we pursue.	
2 minutes	Clarification	[Say] The objective is: To develop an anger management plan. [Say] Today we will: • Draw a symbol of anger • Play a game related to recognizing anger • Brainstorm ways to manage physical symptoms, thoughts and behaviours of anger • Develop a personal anger management plan [Ask] Are we good to go?	Yes.

5 minutes	Warm-up	[Do] Distribute markers and paper. [Say] Choose a coloured marker and draw a symbol to represent the feeling of anger on this blank sheet of paper. Share your drawing and explanation with the group. Say where you experience the symptoms of anger in your body.	Personal response. Example: Colour of red, felt in neck and shoulders, and head due to hot thoughts.
7 minutes	Experience	[Say] I have provided an outline on the flipchart (whiteboard) for the game we will play related to experiencing anger. We will divide into two teams. Each team will take turns choosing a row and column point value. Once it is chosen, I will read the corresponding clue. The team will then decide if the anger clue is an example of a physical symptom, thought or behaviour related to anger. Please answer in the form of a question: What is a physical symptom? What is a thought? What is behaviour? [Do] Refer to: **Game template and resource for therapist/facilitator.** Facilitate game until all sections have been answered and discussed.	Learners participate in the game.

(continued)

Table 3.2 Cont.

Time frame	Learning stage	Facilitator	Expected learner response
5 minutes	Reflection	[Do] Provide handout: **Anger game: Answers.**	Yes/no, possibly section C for 50 points as it is the only constructive action mentioned in the game
		[Ask] Were there any examples or clues provided that were a surprise for you in that they were related to anger?	
		[Ask] Which of these examples have you experienced? Are there any physical symptoms, thoughts or behaviours that you would like to add?	Personal responses
		[Say] Write out your personal anger response in the space provided on the handout.	Learners complete individually
5 minutes	Generalization	[Ask] How do examples such as negative thoughts, fast breaths, closing down or raising our voice impact self and others when we are angry? Can you explain your answers?	Negative and distorted thoughts fuel anger and intense emotions, fast breaths make it hard to think clearly and speeds the heart rate, closing down does not respect oneself, raising voice does not respect the other person so communication can break down.

12 minutes	Application	[Do] Provide handout: **Strategies for changing thoughts, behaviours and physical symptoms of anger.** [Say] Recognizing we are angry is the first step in managing the emotion. Once we recognize what we are experiencing, we can choose to take action to manage it. Here are lists of constructive strategies for managing the experience of anger. Please read through the lists and choose two that are of interest. Then define at least one action specifically. For example: The strategy of exercise can be defined as, "Take a 15-minute brisk walk to decrease energy."	Learners complete worksheet individually.
20 minutes	Evaluation	[Do] Provide handout: **Anger management plan.** [Say] Consider a personal situation related to anger emotions that you would like to find strategies for managing. Choose four constructive anger management strategies that you could use to manage anger symptoms, like reframing a critical thought and replacing a destructive behaviour. Define each strategy as a specific action you could take to manage the anger experience. Then name your personal responsibilities for following the anger management plan. Complete your plan by including a support person you could share your plan with.	Given game, lecture, discussion, practice and feedback; The learner will develop an anger management plan; To the extent that all in writing, four action steps are identified and two personal responsibilities are named; As evaluated by self, peers and therapist/facilitator.

(continued)

Table 3.2 Cont.

Time frame	Learning stage	Facilitator	Expected learner response
		[Say] If comfortable to do so, you can share a brief overview of your answers with the large group.	
1 minute	Wrap up	[Ask] Are there any questions?	Personal response.
		[Do] Thank everyone for coming and participating.	

Reference

Greenberger, D., & Padesky, C. (2016). *Mind over mood: Change how you feel by changing the way you think:* (2nd ed.). New York, NY: Guilford Press

References for Handouts

McKay, M., & Rogers, P. (2000). *The anger control workbook.* Oakland, CA. New Haringer Publications.

3.3 Choosing Occupations for Distress Tolerance and Resilience

LEARNING POINT

Calling on our strengths and coping mechanisms in moments of distress is an important component of regulating emotions. Preplanning ensures items or activities for managing distress are available for use.

LEARNING OBJECTIVE

Given list of coping options, rating scale for mood intensity, lecture, discussion, practice and feedback;

The learner will assemble a first aid kit for emotional comfort;

To the extent that a prescribed worksheet is completed, three physical items are collected, and a commitment is made to use the named items when need is identified;

As evaluated by self, peers and therapist/facilitator.

MATERIALS

Flipchart or whiteboard, markers, highlighters, various items for distress tolerance (puzzle pages, colouring, gum, stress balls, etc.)

HANDOUTS

- Activities with a sensory focus
- Emotional first aid: Items and actions
- Rating tool for mood levels
- My first aid kit for emotional comfort

Table 3.3 Choosing Occupations for Distress Tolerance and Resilience

Time frame	Learning stage	Facilitator	Expected learner response
3 minutes	Orientation	[Say] Welcome, etc. [Say] Managing distress using our strengths and constructive coping strategies can make a positive difference in our ability to handle difficult emotions and distress (Linehan, 1993). Having items or activities readily available makes it easier to choose constructive options.	
2 minutes	Clarification	[Say] The objective is: To assemble a comfort kit/ resource [Say] Today we will: • Brainstorm activities with a sensory focus • Review options for tolerating distressing emotions • Set up a rating tool to define mood levels • Complete a coping plan when need is identified [Ask] Are we good to go?	Yes.
5 minutes	Warm-up	[Do] Provide handout: **Activities with a sensory focus.**	

		[Say] I have listed the five senses as categories. Let's brainstorm two activities that promote pleasant sensory activity for each of the categories.	Learners suggest options in large group.
7 minutes	Experience	[Do] Provide handout: **Emotional first aid: Items and actions**.	
		[Say] Here is a list of items and actions that may help to manage distressing emotions. Read through the list and highlight three to five items/ actions that you have used in the past to help calm yourself. Share your answers.	Learners complete handout individually and share with large group.
5 minutes	Reflection	[Ask] Name two items or activities from the list that you have readily available for your use? What is one new idea you think would be interesting to try?	Personal responses
		[Ask] What is one activity that could calm you if you were anxious or angry? What is one activity that could stimulate you if your mood or energy is low?	Anxious/angry – music, walking, etc.; Low energy – stretching, brush hair, etc.
13 minutes	Generalization	[Say] When we are distressed, it is helpful to understand why our emotional responses and behaviours make sense when put in context of our life and of the moment (Linehan, 1993).	

(continued)

Table 3.3 Cont.

Time frame	Learning stage	Facilitator	Expected learner response
		[Ask] What is a behaviour that you do when in distress that is less constructive? What role does that behaviour play?	Personal responses. Example: Ruminating on negative events may make us feel that we are acting on the problem by trying to solve it. This sense of taking action towards a situation that is distressing to us will relieve some distress in the short term. The reality is usually that we are not solving the problem in that moment.
		[Do] Provide handout: **Rating tool for mood levels**. Read introduction. [Say] You can use this chart as a guide to recognize different levels of distress. Personalize your chart by choosing colours, symbols, thoughts and actions to represent different mood levels.	Learners complete the chart individually.

12 minutes	Application	[Do] Provide handout: **My first aid kit for emotional comfort**. Read the opening paragraph. [Say] Work through the sections on the handout. If stuck for ideas, you may ask suggestions from the large group.	Learners complete handout individually.
11 minutes	Evaluation	[Do] Show the learners the various items for distress tolerance (puzzle pages, colouring, gum, stress balls, etc.) [Say] Refer to the section on the last handout that asks, "Name three items I need to gather or prepare for my kit?" Take time now to gather those items. For example: You can look up a song lyric on your personal electronic device or choose from various items on display that may help you. [Say] Make a commitment to the group regarding one action you will take to put your comfort kit ideas into practice when the need is identified.	Given list of coping options, rating scale for mood intensity, lecture, discussion, practice and feedback; The learner will assemble a first aid kit for emotional comfort; To the extent that a prescribed worksheet is completed, three physical items are collected, and a commitment is made to use the named items when need is identified; As evaluated by self, peers and therapist/facilitator.

(continued)

Table 3.3 Cont.

Time frame	Learning stage	Facilitator	Expected learner response
2 minutes	Wrap up	[Ask] Are there any questions? [Do] Thank everyone for coming and participating.	Personal response.

Reference

Linehan, M., (1993). *Skills training manual for treating borderline personality disorder* (1st ed.). New York, NY: Guilford Press.

References for Handouts

Canadian Armed Forces. (2017). *Road to mental readiness*. Canada. www.google.com/search?sxsrf=ALeKk02Q-gshsSmnJ6rpGYUP115N5LEFTQ:1612718577677&source=univ&tbm=isch&q=canadian+armed+forces+road+to+mental+readiness+self+awareness+colour+chart+colour+chart&sa = X&ved=2ahUKEwjRlsfvpNjuAhXyYN8KHeryC4IQjkEegQIBhAB&biw=1913&bih=902.

Linehan, M. (1993). *Skills training manual for treating borderline personality disorder* (1st ed.). New York, NY: Guilford Press.

Safewards.net. (2010). Calm down methods. London: UK. Safewards.net/images/pdf/Calm-Down-Methods-website-download.pdf

Mai, S. (1987). The Mai color glossary: Instructional manual for an art therapy assessment technique. Ottawa: S.E. Mai. www.worldcat.org/title/mai-color-glossary-instructional-manual-for-an-art-therapy-assessment-technique/oclc/24283882.

3.4 Suicide Safety Plan for Occupational Engagement and Recovery (SSP-OEAR)

Note to facilitator: It is recommended that the facilitator have training in recognizing warning signs, risks factors and protective factors for suicidality, and in counselling to reduce lethal means. It is also recommended that the client have some basic knowledge and skill in coping strategies such as assertive communication, recognizing and managing negative thoughts, recognizing stress exhaustion symptoms, and the benefit of health routines for resilience. For further modules related to these named coping strategies, see the resource: McNamara & Straathof (2017). *Coping strategies to promote occupational engagement and recovery: A program manual for occupational therapists and other care providers.* Upon completion of the SSP-OEAR, a follow up contact is recommended with the client to ensure that supports have been contacted and that the safety plan has been shared with them, **and** that the lethal means have been disposed of as appropriate.

LEARNING POINT

Having a safety plan to follow when suicidal ideation, planning or actions occur will increase one's sense of control and promote safety.

LEARNING OBJECTIVE

Given review of sample, discussion, practice and feedback;
The learner will construct a suicide safety plan,
To the extent that all in writing and with prescribed template, a personal mission statement, warning signs and positive coping strategies are identified, and a verbal commitment is made to share the plan with a support person and to reduce access to lethal means;
As evaluated by self and therapist/facilitator.

MATERIALS

Cards with local crisis line number that can be stored in wallet (optional).

HANDOUTS

- Suicide safety plan for occupational engagement and recovery (SSP-OEAR) – sample
- Suicide safety plan for occupational engagement and recovery (SSP-OEAR)
- Mini suicide safety plan – Wallet size cards (various options are pre-cut cut for presentation)

Table 3.4 Suicide Safety Plan for Occupational Engagement and Recovery (SSP-OEAR)

Time frame	Learning stage	Facilitator	Expected learner response
3 minutes	Orientation	[Say] Welcome, etc. [Say] Suicidal thoughts can be distressing. Past suicide behaviours can be a predictor for future suicide behaviours. Having a safety plan to follow when suicidal ideas, planning or self-harm actions occur will increase one's sense of control, promote safety and reduce risk of suicide (Stanley & Brown, 2012).	
2 minutes	Clarification	[Say] The objective is: To construct a suicide safety plan [Say] Today we will: • Review a sample suicide safety plan • Compare the plan to methods you have used to manage suicide risk • Write a personal suicide safety plan and decide how it will be put to use. [Ask] Are we good to go?	Yes.

Time frame	Learning stage	Facilitator	Expected learner response
3 minutes	Warm-up	[Say] If a community is aware a possible crisis can happen, like flood or tornado, they will often construct an emergency preparedness plan. [Ask] How might an emergency preparedness plan help in managing a crisis? (Option: [Ask] What would you need to know or do to keep you and your family safe from a house fire? Then relate the learner's response to general information about dealing with a crisis and promoting safety). [Ask] What is the benefit of doing the plan before the crisis hits?	They would know warning signs, supplies to manage the crisis are in place, less chaos in crisis, there is a plan to follow, they know who is responsible for what action, etc. Effort can be put into carrying out the plan in the crisis, rather than trying to develop it. It is difficult to make a plan when emotions are running high, easier to follow when you already know what to do, and when others know how they can help.

(continued)

Table 3.4 Cont.

		[Say] A suicide safety plan is a type of emergency preparedness plan.	
4 minutes	Experience	[Do] Provide handout: **SSP-OEAR – sample** (Straathof, in press).	
		[Do] Read through the sample plan together.	
		[Say] Highlight or underline any parts or key words that stand out for you.	Learners highlight key points.
4 minutes	Reflection	[Ask] What is your gut reaction to the layout of this plan?	Personal response (emphasize feeling words). Some may feel anxious, some may feel interested, etc.
		[Ask] How is this safety plan similar to strategies you have used to manage suicide risk? How is it different?	Personal responses such as: Includes warning signs, contact numbers for support services, etc. Differences may be that other plans have less detail.
		[Ask] What is one thing you like about this plan?	Personal response.

Time frame	Learning stage	Facilitator	Expected learner response
7 minutes	Generalization	[Ask] What are the benefits versus the risks of having a suicide safety plan? Why?	Benefit: having a plan may be easier to follow in a stress situation Risk: It may be stressful to complete the plan, may be uncomfortable to share with others.
		[Ask] Why is it important to name your responsibility in using the plan and how your supports could help you?	Everyone plays a part in the safety plan, the person in crisis needs to alert the others and has a say in what could be most helpful from others.
		[Ask] Why is it helpful to reduce or limit access to lethal means?	This could delay suicide actions when emotions are running high or reduce impulsive behaviours. May provide a reminder to ask for help when in crisis.
		[Say] Once in crisis, it can be difficult to follow a plan. We need to consider those barriers impacting follow through in designing a suicide safety plan.	

(*continued*)

Table 3.4 Cont.

		Personal response (example: A barrier could be remembering to use the plan and a strategy could be to put a picture of the plan on personal cell phone or carry a mini plan in personal wallet)
	[Ask] What might be a barrier to implementing a suicide safety plan? How could the barrier you named be overcome?	
Application 20 to 30 minutes	[Do] Provide handout: **SSP-OEAR (front and back).** [Say] Using the template, create your own Suicide Safety Plan. I can assist you if needed. Share it with me when you are finished. (Note: It is often helpful here if the facilitator/therapist offers to capture the ideas from the learner in writing using the template. Remember to use the learner's own words. Remain present for the completion to coach as needed). [Say] **Sometimes in a crisis, it can be helpful to have a mini suicide safety plan to refer to that highlights key points. This can be stored in your wallet or on your phone.**	Learners complete the exercise with support from facilitator as needed. All sections of the safety plan are filled in.

Time frame	Learning stage	Facilitator	Expected learner response
		[Do] Distribute **Mini suicide safety plan – Wallet size cards**. Allow the learner to choose a style that they prefer.	Learner chooses a preferred mini plan and completes the sections.
		[Ask] How would you rate your confidence in using your safety plan from 1 to 10 – 1 being not confident at all and 10 being extremely confident?	Personal response (note to facilitator – look for a score of 7 or higher; if less than 7, work with the learner to increase level of confidence by adjusting the plan).
		[Ask] Would you add anything to your safety plan that would boost your confidence in using the plan to a confidence score of 8 or higher?	
4 minutes	Evaluation	[Say] Name a support you would be willing to share your plan with. Make a commitment to let your supports (personal or professional) know you have a safety plan in the next 24 hours and then set a time to review the safety plan with them. State how you would get a copy of the plan to your supports. If you have strategies to reduce or limit lethal means, state your plan clearly and the actions you would need from your support to ensure this is carried out. If you need to dispose of items, it is recommended that you **not** handle the items for lethal means, but that you have someone to dispose of them for you.	Given review of sample suicide safety plan, discussion, practice and feedback; The learner will construct a suicide safety plan; To the extent that all in writing and with prescribed template, a personal mission statement, warning signs and positive coping strategies are identified; and a verbal commitment is made to share the plan with a support

(continued)

		person and to reduce access to lethal means; As evaluated by self and therapist/facilitator.
	[Ask] How many copies of your safety plan would you like to have for yourself and to share with others? [Ask] Where would you leave this plan to promote the application? Would you like to take a picture of it to have on your phone? Would you like it scanned to your electronic health record or paper chart?	
3 minutes	Wrap up	[Ask] Do you have any questions?	Personal response.

Adapted and reprinted with permission from CAOT Publications ACE. For more information about the development of the SSP-OEAR, see Straathof (in press).

References

Stanley, B., & Brown, G. (2012). Safety planning intervention: A brief intervention to mitigate suicide risk. Cognitive and Behavioral Practice. 19(2). 256–264.

Straathof, T. (in press). Suicide safety plans: Content and process for implementation. *Occupational Therapy Now*.

References for Handouts

Crowley, P., Carmichael, D., Marshall, C., & Murphy, S. (31 May 2019). Safety planning for suicide prevention: A scoping review. Canadian Association of Occupational Therapists Conference, Niagara Falls, ON.

McNamara, M., & Straathof, T. (2017). *Coping strategies to promote occupational engagement and recovery: A program manual for occupational therapists and other care providers.* Ottawa, Ontario: CAOT.

Stanley, B., & Brown, G. (2012). Safety Planning Intervention: A Brief Intervention to Mitigate Suicide Risk. *Cognitive and Behavioral Practice, 19(2), 256–264.*

Straathof, T. (in press). Suicide safety plans: Content and process for implementation. *Occupational Therapy Now*.

3 Change Body Response to Stress

3.1 Behaviour Activation to Assist with Initiating Occupation

Behaviour experiment

PRE-TEST

Choose a number between 1 and 10, and circle the number that best represents your mood at this time. 1 = "the worst," while 10 = "the best"

(the worst) 1   2   3   4   5   6   7   8   9   10   (the best)

Perform behaviour experiment by following instruction of facilitator.

POST-TEST

Choose a number between 1 and 10, and circle the number that best represents your mood at this time. 1 = "the worst," while 10 = "the best"

(the worst) 1   2   3   4   5   6   7   8   9   10 (the best)

What did you notice with your score? _____

What three ideas in this experiment were used in an attempt to boost mood? (Summarize based on large group discussion)

1. M_____
2. P_____
3. M_____

Write one reason for each idea above that explains why it impacts mood and energy.

1.

2.

3.

Getting unstuck

When individuals are depressed, stressed or have serious mental illness, they may withdraw from others and their daily routines. This inactivity may lead to more negative thoughts and avoidance, which in turn takes away opportunity for pleasant activity and a sense of accomplishment (Krupa et al., 2010). Certain types of activity involvement can boost mood and self-esteem, and improve anxiety.

Four types of effective activity involvement (Greenberger & Padesky, 2016) include:

- Movement
- Pleasure
- Mastery
- Overcoming avoidance

Movement (check with your physician before engaging in strenuous activity)*

- Physical activity and movement can reduce depression (Biddle & Mutrie, 2001).
- Physical activity can reduce tension from the stress response (Bourne, 2020).
- Physical activity can improve health (US Department of Health and Human Services, 1996).
- The interaction of mind and body during activity can stimulate neuron growth, stimulate right-brain function, and bypass rigid patterns of thinking (Gabora, 2002; Perrin, 2001).

Pleasure

- Pleasure may include sports, leisure, or playful actions such as humour, curiosity, or interaction with others (Hutton, 2008).
- Pleasure fosters motivation, socialization, energy, communication, flexible thinking and is important for health and wellness (Royeen, 1997).

Mastery

- Activity can create hope, a sense of control of health, and builds confidence (Krupa, 2010).
- Activity involvement can develop knowledge, skills, creative expression, and can lead to interaction and contribution (Krupa, 2010).

References

Biddle S., & Mutrie, N. (2001). Psychology of physical activity: Determinants, well-being and interventions. *Medicine & Science in Sports & Exercise.* Routledge, London. doi:10.4324/9780203019320 Source: OAI.

Bourne, E. (2020). *The anxiety and phobia workbook* (7th ed.). Oakland, CA: New Harbinger Publications. Cole, M. B. (2008).

Gabora, I. (2002). Cognitive mechanisms underlying the creative process. In T. Hewett & T. Kavanaugh (Eds.), *Proceedings of the Fourth International Conference on Creativity and Cognition, 13–16 October* (pp. 126–133). Leicestershire, UK: Loughborough University.

Greenberger, D., & Padesky, C. (2016). *Mind over mood: Change how you feel by changing the way you think*: (2nd ed.). New York, NY: Guilford Press.

Hutton, D. (2008). Play. In J. Creek and L. Lougher (Eds.), *Occupational therapy and mental health, fourth edition.* (pp. 345–358). Philadelphia: Churchill Livingstone Elsevier.

Krupa, T., Edgelow, M., Chen, S., Mieras, C., Almas, A., Perry, A., & Bransfield, M. (2010). *Action over inertia: Addressing the activity-health needs of individuals with serious mental illness.* Ottawa, ON: CAOT publications ACE.

Perrin, T. (2001). Don't despise the fluffy bunny: A reflection from practice. *The British Journal of Occupational Therapy, 64,* 129–134. doi:10.1177/030802260106400304.

Royeen, C. (1997). Play as occupation and as an indicator in health. In B. Chandler (Ed.). The essence of play: A child's occupation. American Occupational Therapy Association, Bethesda, Maryland. (pp. 1–14).

US Department of Health and Human Services (1996). Physical activity and health: A report of the Surgeon General (Executive summary). Superintendent of documents. Pittsburgh, PA.

Overcoming avoidance

The following three strategies can help when feeling stuck, anxious or disinterested (Greenberger & Padesky, 2016).

1. Timed tasks – *Follow the 5-minute rule.* Give yourself only 5 minutes to work on a task. Once the 5 minutes is up, you get full credit. Likely you will keep going with the task that you have started. You can adapt the time from 2 to 10 minutes, or at your discretion. Try this for exercise, emails or sorting papers, etc.
2. Graded tasks – *Break task into small steps.* By taking a small action towards a task, inertia may be broken. When we are lying in our bed or in front of a screen for example, it takes greater effort to become active. Once a task is started, it is easier to keep going. Try this to get up in the morning. Instead of saying "I can't face my day," say "I will sit up, I will put my feet on the floor, I will brush my teeth." Once you are up and moving, the other activities may come a little easier.
3. Prediction logs – *Prediction verses actual scores.* Predict how difficult something will be to do and rate this difficulty on a scale from 1 to 10. Then carry out the task, and rate how difficult it actually was to do. Likely the prediction for difficulty will be higher than the actual score. You can also use a positive predictor, such as how much enjoyment you will get out of doing the task. In this case, your prediction score may be lower than the actual score, because low mood impacts the belief that you will get pleasure from the activity.

Example for prediction log: A young man who became quite isolated gave this a try. He decided he would spend an hour with a friend watching a sporting event on TV. He predicted he would experience a pleasure of 4/10. After doing the activity, he rated it as a 7/10. Several friends came to the event and he was pleased he could join in some of the conversation around the event.

Action initiative

1. Choose a task you have difficulty doing in your day or that you have been avoiding and write it in the space below.

2. Choose one strategy to help you get unstuck with your task and circle your choice.

   Small steps   5-minute rule   Prediction log

3. Define how you will put this strategy into action in the next 24 hours in the space below.

Reference

Greenberger, D., & Padesky, C. (2016). *Mind over mood: Change how you feel by changing the way you think*: (2nd ed.). New York, NY: Guilford Press.

3.2 Anger Management Strategies for Constructive Action

Game template and resource for therapist/facilitator

Anger game template – Copy this template on flipchart or whiteboard

	50 points	100 points	150 points
A			
B			
C			
D			

Clues for the game follow outlining physical symptoms, thoughts and behaviours related to anger. Learners provide answers in the form of a question. If correct, place team name in the blank template space.

Example: Team A chooses Row A for 50 points
Facilitator reads clue: Raised, loud voice
Learner answers: What is behaviour?
Team A is correct and gets 50 points, then play switches to team B.

	50 points	*100 points*	*150 points*
A	Raised, loud voice *(Answer: What is behaviour?)*	I should have dealt with this problem earlier and now it is too late *(Answer: What is a thought?)*	Feeling warm or flushed *(Answer: What is a symptom?)*
B	Muscle tension *(Answer: What is a symptom?)*	Closing down and not speaking to others *(Answer: What is behaviour?)*	She is so selfish not to agree with my requests *(Answer: What is a thought?)*
C	Taking time to write out what you need or want to ask of the other person *(Answer: What is behaviour?)*	I will hurt or offend this person if I say I am angry *(Answer: What is a thought?)*	Blaming others or self for the problem *(Answer: What is behaviour?)*
D	Increased heart rate *(Answer: What is a symptom)*	Quick, short breaths *(Answer: What is a symptom)*	This is not fair *(Answer: What is a thought?)*

Game template and resource for therapist/facilitator (continued)

Instructions for therapist/facilitator:

- Divide group into two teams
- Each person of each team will take a turn to choose a category and point value
- The instructor will read the clue related to row and category point value
- Team member states what it is, in the form of a question (i.e. What is a physical symptom? … a thought? … behaviour?). All clues relate to anger experiences
- If correct, the team member owns the point value and play switches to the other team
- If incorrect, the other team has an opportunity to guess the correct answer, gains the point value and then play goes back to the team that had the incorrect answer
- Play continues until all clues have been provided and correctly answered

Anger game: Answers

	50 points	*100 points*	*150 points*
A	Raised, loud voice (*behaviour*)	I should have dealt with this problem earlier and now it is too late (*thought*)	Feeling warm or flushed (*physical symptom*)
B	Muscle tension (*physical symptom*)	Closing down and not speaking to others (*behaviour*)	She is so selfish not to agree with my requests (*thought*)
C	Taking time to write out what you need or want to ask of the other person (*behaviour*)	I will hurt or offend this person if I say I am angry (*thought*)	Blaming others or self for the problem (*behaviour*)
D	Increased heart rate (*physical symptom*)	Quick, short breaths (*physical symptom*)	This is not fair (*thought*)

Personal anger response: Write your answers in the space below.

• What happens to me when I feel angry?

• Physical symptoms:

• Thoughts:

• Behaviours:

• Situations that trigger emotions related to anger:

Strategies for changing thoughts, behaviours and physical symptoms of anger

Thoughts: Look for evidence of thought distortions or negative thoughts that may intensify the emotions. Words such as should, shouldn't, always, never, unfair, or words that imply blame may be a distortion in thinking. Try the following strategies:

- Recognize thought distortions or negative thoughts
- Reframe the thought to one that is positive, neutral or compassionate
- Remind yourself that you have a right to express your thoughts and feelings in a calm and respectful manner
- Remind yourself that you can control your thoughts and actions, not those of others
- Express your feelings and needs calmly to keep communication open

Behaviours: Behaviours may be constructive or destructive. In managing anger, it is important to choose behaviour that is respectful to you and to others. However, being respectful does not imply that you give in to others needs and wants while sacrificing your own needs and wants. There may be room for compromise or realistic consequences (McKay & Rogers, 2000). Try the following strategies:

- Take responsibility for your anger
- Burn off the energy related to anger
- Feel the emotion, and accept that it is as valid as any other feeling
- Write out the thinking related to the anger
- Make a responsible decision about what action, if any, that you want to take
- Keep communication open with others regarding your thoughts, feelings and needs
- Have discussions related to anger when you and the other person are calm and likely to listen
- Be prepared to listen to the other person's perspective

Physical symptoms: Find ways to deepen the breathing, reduce the heart rate and muscle tension, and cool the body. Try the following strategies:

- Deep breathing
- Exercise
- Relax/distract
- Cool the body

Choose two examples in total from the above strategies that are of interest to you. Highlight your choices in some way. Define the strategy as a specific action. For

Strategies for changing thoughts, behaviours and physical symptoms of anger (continued)

example, cooling the body can be defined as: I will sit down for 5 minutes and slowly drink an iced water.

1. _____

2. _____

Reference

McKay, M., & Rogers, P. (2000). *The anger control workbook*. Oakland, CA: New Harbinger Publications.

Anger management plan

A. Name a personal situation related to anger emotions and write it in the space below. Provide details about your thoughts and behaviour related to the situation. Define the emotions more specifically with anger words such as frustration, furious or enraged.

B. Name four constructive strategies that you could use related to this personal situation. Define each strategy as a specific action in the spaces in the table.

Strategy	Specific action
Example: Change negative thinking	I will remind myself that I have a right to respectfully let the person know how their behaviour made me feel
1.	
2.	
3.	
4.	

C. State how you could demonstrate personal responsibility for managing anger and write it in the space below. Example: I am responsible for using respectful communication.

D. Who would you share your anger management plan with? How would you like that person to support you? Example: I will share my plan with my brother and ask him to walk with me so I can cool down.

My support person:

How my support person could help me:

3.3 Choosing Occupations for Distress Tolerance and Resilience

Activities with a sensory focus

The following five categories are related to our senses of seeing, hearing, smelling, tasting and touching. Engaging in pleasant sensory activities is one way to manage distressing emotions (Linehan, 1993). Please name two ideas for each category that can be used to soothe the senses.

Sight: Example: Flowers

1. _____
2. _____

Sound: Example: Waterfall

1. _____
2. _____

Smell: Example: Vanilla

1. _____
2. _____

Taste: Example: Mint

1. _____
2. _____

Touch: Example: Soft socks

1. _____
2. _____

Reference

Linehan, M. (1993). *Skills training manual for treating borderline personality disorder* (1st ed.). New York, NY: Guilford Press.

Emotional first aid: Items and actions

This list includes items and actions that may help to manage distressing emotions. Read through the list and highlight three to five items that you have used in the past week to help calm yourself. Put a star beside one new idea you think would be interesting to try.

Sensory stimulation				
Warm towel	Music	Colouring	Ice	Soft blanket
Cold cloth	Walking	Snack	Cold water	Shower/bath
Animal videos	Lotion	Brush hair	Herbal tea	Cuddle toy
Scented markers	Feather	Watch nature	Plasticine	Fan self
Nature sounds	Stretching	Fold clothes	Magazines	Mint
Song lyrics	Dance	Make bed	Gum	Stress balls

Other: _____

Challenge/Mastery	
Craft project (origami, weaving, sanding, knitting, etc.)	Collage
Writing (card, poetry, story, etc.)	Positive statements
Puzzles (word search, Sudoku, etc.)	Colour

Other: _____

Social interaction		
Call friend/family	Walk together	Ask for assistance
Initiate conversation	Play a game	Smile
Act of kindness	Share a joke	Compliment someone

Other: _____

Movement and/or Relaxation			
Box breathing	Five senses	Yoga	Exercise/Stretching

Other: _____

Rating tool for mood levels

Introduction: A distress experience relates to moods in the mad, sad or fear families. There can often be overlap in these families of emotions. Another way to define level of distress (combined physical and emotional distress) could be by using a colour chart or a number scale.

Personalize the chart below to define what happens to you at different mood levels. Choose a colour and/or symbol to represent levels of mood intensity. Fill in situations, thoughts and behaviours related to each level.

Mood level (colour)	Mood–symbol or number scale (1 to 10) (Optional)	Situations that trigger mood intensity or neutrality	Examples of my thoughts at each level	Examples of my behaviours at each level
High distress				
Moderate distress				
Neutral, calm, relaxed, optimistic				

Inspired by: Canadian Armed Forces, 2017; Safewards.net, 2010; Mai, 1987)

References

Canadian Armed Forces. (2017). *Road to mental readiness*. Canada.

Mai, S. (1987). The Mai color glossary: Instructional manual for an art therapy assessment technique. Ottawa: S.E. Mai.

Safewards.net. (2010). Calm down methods. London: UK.

My first aid kit for emotional comfort

Now that you have defined the different mood levels, you will be better able to recognize when emotional first aid is needed. Refer to the suggested items and actions from the previous handout. Choose ideas for your first aid kit that could provide emotional comfort and move you towards the neutral zone when need is identified.

List two actions I can take and two items I can use to manage HIGH distress:

High distress: Actions	High distress: Items

List two actions I can take and two items I can use to manage MODERATE distress:

Moderate distress: Actions	Moderate distress: Items

Name three items I would need to gather or prepare to have ready in my kit (e.g. lyrics for a song, a colouring page, a wellness routine, etc.)

1. _____
2. _____
3. _____

Describe my strengths that will help me use the first aid kit to comfort me in the space below.

What will I need to ask of others to assist me in managing my distress?

How will I use this comfort kit in the next 24 hours?

3.4 Suicide safety plan for occupational engagement and recovery (SSP-OEAR)

Suicide safety plan for occupational engagement and recovery (SSP-OEAR) – sample

Suicide thoughts, planning and actions can increase risk of injury and death; safety plans outline steps to take for reducing suicide risk (Stanley & Brown, 2012).

Name: **Date**:

MISSION STATEMENT

What is my reason to live? What brings me meaning and purpose? *My mission is to take care of myself so I can also take care of my family.*

WORDS OF OTHERS

Why others appreciate me, and say I am important and valuable.
   "You are the kindest person I know!" – Aunt Mary; my spouse enjoys my artwork

WARNING SIGNS OF SUICIDE RISK

Triggers: *Family gatherings with alcohol present*
Negative thoughts: *"They would be better off without me."*
Emotions: *Guilt, anxiety, hopelessness*
Physical symptoms: *Not sleeping, low energy, crying*
Actions: *Isolating, staying in bed, not eating, stopping my medication*

COPING STRATEGIES

I can take these steps when warning signs are present to stay safe:

A balanced thought: *My family and friends value me.*
To manage emotions: *Take deep, slow breaths. Talk with my friend.*
To manage physical symptoms: *Go for a walk. Listen to upbeat music. Take a warm bath.*
Constructive actions: *Put alarm on phone as a reminder for medication. Read. Do crafts.*
A social interaction for distraction: *Invite Aunt Mary for coffee. Go to the museum with Jim.*
An act of kindness I can do: *Walk my neighbour's dog. Donate two items to the food bank.*

How can I make my environment safe? – Remove lethal means. Add healthy means.

I will only keep a small amount of necessary over-the-counter medication at home.
I will only keep the necessary number of sharps, and I will keep them in a secure space.

Name my responsibility in using this safety plan:

I will follow the plan. I will keep a healthy sleep routine and meal routine.

Name two people I will share the plan with and state what support they could provide:

1. *Jim (significant other): (phone number): Assist me to hospital if needed.*
2. *Margaret (counsellor): (phone number): Assist me to resolve the crisis.*

(Continued on next page)

Suicide safety plan for occupational engagement and recovery (SSP-OEAR) – sample (continued)

Name: *Date*:

Supports (name) and health care services	Phone number/location
Emergency contact:	
Emergency response services:	911
Crisis line:	
Emergency department:	
Family physician:	
Psychiatrist:	
Counsellor/sponsor/other:	
Pharmacy:	

Healthy lifestyle checklist for review (McNamara & Straathof, 2017)
(*Check off two to three activities to prioritize for maintaining health, wellness and resilience*)

- ☐ Eating regular nutritious meals
- ☐ Maintaining a healthy sleep routine
- ☐ Exercising regularly
- ☐ Taking medications as prescribed
- ☐ Limiting substance use (alcohol, street drugs, caffeine, other)
- ☐ Keeping in touch with the people who support me
- ☐ Participating in meaningful social and leisure activity
- ☐ Keeping appointments with my doctors and counsellors
- ☐ Using assertive communication
- ☐ Doing deep breathing
- ☐ Encouraging myself with positive or balanced self-talk

Name places where I could keep copies of this plan: *By my bed and on my phone.*

I commit to reviewing my plan (circle 1): daily   weekly   monthly   other

For more information about the development of the SSP-OEAR, see Straathof (in press). Reprinted with permission from CAOT Publications ACE. Adapted from: Crowley, Carmichael, Marshall & Murphy, 2019; Stanley & Brown, 2012.

References

Crowley, P., Carmichael, D., Marshall, C. & Murphy, S. (31 May 2019). Safety planning for suicide prevention: A scoping review. Canadian Association of Occupational Therapists Conference, Niagara Falls, ON.

McNamara, M., & Straathof, T. (2017). *Coping strategies to promote occupational engagement and recovery: A program manual for occupational therapists and other care providers.* Ottawa, ON: CAOT.

Stanley, B., & Brown, G. (2012). Safety planning intervention: A brief intervention to mitigate suicide risk. *Cognitive and Behavioral Practice,* 19(2), 256–264.

Straathof, T. (in press). Suicide safety plans: Content and process for implementation. *Occupational Therapy Now.*

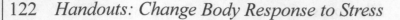

Suicide safety plan for occupational engagement and recovery
(SSP-OEAR)

Suicide thoughts, planning and actions can increase risk of injury and death; safety plans outline steps to take for reducing suicide risk (Stanley & Brown, 2012).

Name: **Date**:

MISSION STATEMENT

What is my reason to live? What brings me meaning and purpose?

WORDS OF OTHERS

Why others appreciate me, and say I am important and valuable**?**

WARNING SIGNS OF SUICIDE RISK

Triggers:
Negative thoughts:
Emotions*:*
Physical symptoms*:*
Actions:

COPING STRATEGIES

I can take these steps when warning signs are present to stay safe:

A balanced thought:
To manage emotions:
To manage physical symptoms:
Constructive actions:
A social interaction for distraction:
An act of kindness I can do:

How can I make my environment safe? – Remove lethal means. Add healthy means.

Name my responsibility in using this safety plan:

Name two people I will share the plan with and state what support they could provide:

1.
2.

(Continued on next page)

Suicide safety plan for occupational engagement and recovery (SSP-OEAR) (continued)

Name: *Date*:

Supports (name) and health care services	Phone number/location
Emergency contact:	
Emergency response services:	911
Crisis line:	
Emergency department:	
Family physician:	
Psychiatrist:	
Counsellor/sponsor/other:	
Pharmacy:	

Healthy Lifestyle checklist for review (McNamara & Straathof, 2017)

(*Check off two to three activities to prioritize for maintaining health, wellness and resilience*)

- ☐ Eating regular nutritious meals
- ☐ Maintaining a healthy sleep routine
- ☐ Exercising regularly
- ☐ Taking medications as prescribed
- ☐ Limiting substance use (alcohol, street drugs, caffeine, other)
- ☐ Keeping in touch with the people who support me
- ☐ Participating in meaningful social and leisure activity
- ☐ Keeping appointments with my doctors and counsellors
- ☐ Using assertive communication
- ☐ Doing deep breathing
- ☐ Encouraging myself with positive or balanced self-talk

Name places where I could keep copies of this plan:

I commit to reviewing my plan (circle 1): daily   weekly   monthly   other

For more information about the development of the SSP-OEAR, see Straathof (in press). Reprinted with permission from CAOT Publications ACE. Adapted from: Crowley, Carmichael, Marshall & Murphy, 2019; Stanley & Brown, 2012.

References

Crowley, P., Carmichael, D., Marshall, C. & Murphy, S. (31 May 2019). Safety planning for suicide prevention: A scoping review. Canadian Association of Occupational Therapists Conference, Niagara Falls, ON.

McNamara, M., & Straathof, T. (2017). *Coping strategies to promote occupational engagement and recovery: A program manual for occupational therapists and other care providers.* Ottawa, ON: CAOT.

Stanley, B., & Brown, G. (2012). Safety planning intervention: A brief intervention to mitigate suicide risk. *Cognitive and Behavioral Practice, 19*(2), 256–264.

Straathof, T. (in press). Suicide safety plans: Content and process for implementation. *Occupational Therapy Now.*

Mini suicide safety plan – Wallet size cards (cut and separated)

Mission Statement – My reason to live: **Constructive Coping Strategy:** **Refer to Original Suicide Safety Plan Call 911 or Call Crisis Line:**	**Supports (Personal and Professional)** 1.Name: Phone Number: 2. Name: Phone Number: 3. Name: Phone Number:
My reason to live: **Quote from others:** **Constructive Coping Strategy:** **Refer to Original Safety Plan Call 911 or Call Crisis Line:**	**Supports (Personal and Professional)** 1.Name: Phone Number: 2. Name: Phone Number: 3. Name: Phone Number:
What gives me meaning and purpose? **Why others appreciate me:** **Constructive Coping Strategy:** **Refer to Original Safety Plan Call 911 or Call Crisis Line:**	**Supports (Personal and Professional)** 1.Name: Phone Number: 2. Name: Phone Number: 3. Name: Phone Number:
Mission Statement – My reason to live: **Helpful mantra:** **Helpful Coping Strategy:** **Refer to Original Safety Plan Call 911 or Call Crisis Line:**	**Supports (Family, Friends, Other)** 1.Name: Phone Number: 2. Name: Phone Number: 3. Name: Phone Number:

4 Modules

Change Attitude

4.1 Building On Our Strengths to Aid With Occupation Engagement

LEARNING POINT

Borrowing strategies from those occupations we excel in can build resilience for our occupation challenges.

LEARNING OBJECTIVE

Given warm-up, steps for building resilience, lecture, discussion, practice and feedback;

The learner will identify a symbol;

To the extent that a personal strength is represented and a verbal explanation is provided as to how strategies from the strength occupation will be used to increase success with one occupational challenge;

As evaluated by self, peers and therapist/facilitator.

MATERIALS

Whiteboard or flipchart and markers

DOI: 10.4324/9781003189695-5

HANDOUTS

- Accessing your strengths
- Matching exercise (Max)
- Using strengths to develop resilience
- Symbol of strength

Table 4.1 Building on our strengths to aid with occupation engagement

Time frame	Learning stage	Facilitator	Expected learner response
3 minutes	Orientation	Say] Welcome, etc. [Say] Resilience is not something we are born with, but rather it is learned and developed (Thibeault, 2011). For this to occur, it helps to remember that adaptation is possible and that our strengths from occupation successes can be used for occupation challenges.	
2 minutes	Clarification	[Say] The objective is: To generate a personal symbol of strength. [Say] Today we will: • Identify an area of strength • Create a symbol representing our strengths • Apply our strengths to manage a challenge [Ask] Are we good to go?	Yes.

(continued)

5 minutes	Warm-up	[Do] Provide handout: **Accessing your strengths.** [Say] Choose a strength from the following options: • One personal occupation you do every day • Something you are good at (an interest, a subject) • A positive way in which you are described by others, etc. Share with the group and include one reason why that strength is important to you.	Personal response
3 minutes	Experience	[Do] Return to the next section of the handout: **Accessing your strengths.** [Say] Padesky & Mooney (2012) introduced a process for developing resilience through reflecting on our strengths, constructing a personal model for resilience, applying the model to challenges and then practising our use of the model through behaviour experiments. The process we use today is inspired by their work but is simplified for your use. Let's read through the rest of the handout together.	
10 minutes	Reflection	[Ask] What is your gut reaction to this approach? [Do] Provide handout: **Matching exercise (Max).**	Personal response

Table 4.1 Cont.

Time frame	Learning stage	Facilitator	Expected learner response
		[Say] Here is a sample of what the process would look like with the steps named and the action at each stage outlined. Match the number of the step to the action indicated by a letter. For example: Step 1 matches with the action letter D.	Learners complete the task in pairs. Answers: 1 – D, 2 – C, 3 – E, 4 – B, 5 – A
5 minutes	Generalization	[Ask] What makes the sequence in the process significant?	Identifying resilience in an area of strength provides a foundation to summarize strategies.
		[Ask] What can we discover about someone when his or her occupation remains a priority even when difficulties arise? Why is that?	We can discover personal qualities, characteristics, skills, talents, values, etc. When we put high meaning on an occupation, we can persist despite obstacles.
15 minutes	Application	[Do] Provide handout: **Using strengths to develop resilience.** [Say] Refer to your strength occupation identified during the warm-up to complete this worksheet.	Learners complete the handout individually.

		[Do] Circulate to answer questions and provide coaching. Pay particular attention to the conclusions looking for at least three summarized strategies.	Given warm-up, steps for building resilience, lecture, discussion, practice and feedback; The learner will identify a symbol; To the extent that a personal strength is represented and a verbal explanation is provided as to how strategies from the strength occupation will be used to increase success with one occupational challenge; As evaluated by self, peers and therapist/facilitator.
14 minutes	Evaluation	[Do] Provide handout: **Symbol of strength.** [Say] Let's return to the earlier example of Max. Recall his strength occupation was cleaning the bed sheets. Having a symbol or metaphor to represent our strengths can be a powerful reminder in new and challenging situations. A symbol to represent the strength activity of washing bed sheets weekly could be a pillow with the words "I am strong." The symbol represents being organized, helpful and tidy. The summary of strategies with cleaning was to do small steps, ask for help and make it part of a routine. [Say] Draw a symbol such as an animal, book, movie character or object that represents your personal strengths. Under your symbol, write three personal characteristics associated with your symbol.	

(continued)

Table 4.1 Cont.

Time frame	Learning stage	Facilitator	Expected learner response
		[Say] Identify an occupation challenge in your day where you are struggling and write it in the space provided. [Say] From your handout: Using strengths to develop resilience, choose two strategies from your conclusion that you could apply to stay resilient with your identified occupation challenge.	
3 minutes	Wrap up	[Ask] Are there any questions? [Do] Thank everyone for coming and participating.	Personal response.

Reference

Padesky, C., & Mooney, K. (2012). Strengths-based cognitive-behavioural therapy: A four-step model to build resilience. *Clinical Psychology and Psychotherapy*, 19, 283–290. https://doi.org/10.1002/cpp.1795.
Thibeault, R. (2011) Resilience and maturity. In M. A. McColl (Ed.), *Spirituality and occupational therapy*. Ottawa, ON: CAOT publications ACE.

References for Handouts

Padesky, C., & Mooney, K. (2012). Strengths-based cognitive-behavioural therapy: A four-step model to build resilience. *Clinical Psychology and Psychotherapy*, 19, 283–290. https://doi.org/10.1002/cpp.1795.

4.2 Problem Solving to Address Challenges in Occupations

LEARNING POINT

There is a process to follow for problem solving.

LEARNING OBJECTIVE

Given problem scenario, brainstorming, discussion, practice and feedback;

The learner will demonstrate problem solving;

To the extent that a prescribed sequence is followed, one action is chosen that can be initiated that same day, one resource for assistance is identified, and one strategy to manage emotional challenges is named;

As evaluated by self, peers and therapist/facilitator.

MATERIALS

White board or flipchart and markers

HANDOUTS

- Steps to creative problem solving
- Problem solving worksheet

Table 4.2 Problem solving to address challenges in occupations

Time frame	Learning stage	Facilitator	Expected learner response
3 minutes	Orientation	[Say] Welcome, etc. [Say] When confronted with a specific problem, it can be difficult to identify options and possible solutions. We may feel strong emotions related to not having the answer right away. Knowing a problem-solving process can generate creative options. From these options, a decision can be made to address the problem. Improved satisfaction occurs by taking action to address the challenge, rather than avoiding the challenge.	
2 minutes	Clarification	[Say] The objective is: To demonstrate a problem-solving sequence. [Say] Today we will: • Review a problem scenario • List the steps of problem solving • Link emotions to the various steps • Complete a worksheet related to a personal problem and choose an action that can be taken today [Ask] Are we good to go?	Yes.

5 minutes	Warm-up	[Say] When you are faced with a problem, what is one thing about solving the problem that is difficult for you?	Intense emotions such as feeling overwhelmed, guilt, anxiety; generating ideas to address the problem; procrastination or avoidance, etc.
3 minutes	Experience	[Say] I am going to tell you a story of a problem scenario. *A student in hospital on the mental health unit lost her student card and cannot access her college dorm room. This is worrying her, but she puts off dealing with it. It is now 4 pm in the afternoon and she does not know how or who to contact to help her get into her room. The college is open the following day only and then will close for two weeks over the winter break. It is also during the pandemic so many admin staff work from home and it is unclear if the admin building is open. Her mother is coming from out of town to move her items home. The student is not returning to the program at this time. Her mother does not yet know she is in hospital. The student is planning for discharge the following day. She is thinking, "There is nothing that can be done to get into my room and my mom will be mad." This is increasing her anxiety.*	

(continued)

Table 4.2 Cont.

Time frame	Learning stage	Facilitator	Expected learner response
12 minutes	Reflection	[Ask] What problems exist in this scenario?	Problems: In hospital, student card lost, no access to room, unclear how to contact the school, mother is coming, mother is not aware of hospital admission, negative thoughts.
		[Ask] Which problem does she have some control over?	Trying to contact the school, as it is still open one more day. Changing the negative thought as it is increasing anxiety.
		Which problem do you think is the priority to address?	Personal response.
		[Ask] What feelings did you experience as you listened to the scenario?	Personal response.
11 minutes	Generalization	[Ask] Once the problem is identified, what are next steps in managing the problem? [Do] Record answers on flip chart.	1. Define the problem 2. Brainstorm ideas for options or solutions 3. Choose options 4. Try it out 5. Evaluate level of success

[Do] Provide handout: **Steps to creative problem solving**. Have members take turns reading the information aloud.	
[Say] Compare the handout to the list the group created.	Similarities and differences are noted. Likely to be similar.
[Ask] What are the benefits of including all six steps suggested in the handout? Why?	Sets up structured actions to take and breaks the problem-solving into smaller steps.
[Ask] In the story about the student, what might be three possible options to get access to her room?	Possible answers: E-mail/call the school, go in person to the administration office, contact a fellow student in the same dorm to let her in.
[Ask] What feelings did you experience as you worked through the steps of identifying the student's problem and finding solutions?	Responses may vary from interest, curiosity and anxiety. Frustration when first facing the problem, then satisfaction on deciding an action to take.

(*continued*)

Table 4.2 Cont.

Time frame	Learning stage	Facilitator	Expected learner response
		[Ask] When stuck, what might be helpful to remember? What could you do to coach yourself to find a solution instead of becoming paralyzed by negative self–talk? [Ask] What are the consequences of avoidance or procrastination when faced with a problem?	Encourage yourself, humour, build on ideas, deep breathing, use others' expertise, or follow a problem-solving process. May lead to greater problems such as missing a deadline.
13 minutes	Application	[Do] Provide handout: **Problem solving worksheet.** [Say] Identify a personal problem you are facing today or in the near future. Follow the sequence of steps from 1 to 3 on the worksheet. Write out your ideas and answers to the questions.	Learners complete the worksheet individually.
10 minutes	Evaluation	[Say] From your short list of three options, answer Section 4. Choose the option that seems the best one at this time. State one reason for your choice. [Say] Next, complete Section 5: Try out the option. • Identify one specific action you can take today that fits with the option you chose. • Name a resource that could help you with this problem	Given problem scenario, brainstorming, discussion, practice and feedback; The learner will demonstrate problem solving; To the extent that a prescribed sequence is followed, one action

		• List a positive statement that will help you take action • Identify one strategy you will use if you get stuck or have uncomfortable feelings related to working through the problem [Say] Finally, state how you will evaluate your success with respect to your specific action? [Do] Circulate among the learners and check their work.	is chosen that can be initiated that same day, one resource for assistance is identified, and one strategy to manage emotional challenges is named; As evaluated by self, peers and therapist/facilitator.
1 minute	Wrap up	[Ask] Are there any questions? [Do] Thank everyone for coming and participating.	Personal response.

4.3 Intentional Positive Occupations to Boost Mental Health

LEARNING POINT

Happiness, wellness and resilience are traits that we can develop and nurture through the choices we make in how we occupy our time.

LEARNING OBJECTIVE

Given lecture, key points for resilience, discussion, practice and feedback;

The learner will construct a template for intentional positive occupation;

To the extent that two categories to support resilience are named, each with two entry suggestions and a commitment is made to participate in one activity for happiness and wellness in the next 24 hours;

As evaluated by self, peers and therapist/facilitator.

MATERIALS

Whiteboard or flipchart and markers

HANDOUTS

- Key factors in building resilience, wellness and happiness
- Occupation categories for resilience, wellness and happiness

Table 4.3 Intentional positive occupations to boost mental health

Time frame	Learning stage	Facilitator	Expected learner response
3 minutes	Orientation	[Say] Happiness, wellness and resilience are traits that we can develop and nurture through the choices we make in how we occupy our time. Intentional positive activities can be used as a coping strategy to mitigate things like rumination and loneliness (Layous, Chancellor & Lyubomirsky, 2014). Research has also found that engaging in positive occupation can boost positive emotions, thoughts and behaviours, in addition to satisfying our needs (Lyubomirsky & Layous, 2013).	
2 minutes	Clarification	[Say] The objective is: To choose intentional, positive occupation. [Say] Today we will: • Outline key points in building resilience • Provide categories for occupations to support resilience, wellness and happiness • Build a template to track our choices for positive occupation	

(continued)

Table 4.3 Cont.

Time frame	Learning stage	Facilitator	Expected learner response
10 minutes	Warm-up	[Say] Name a positive way you have occupied yourself in the past week and tell us the impact it had on your emotions, thoughts and behaviours?	Learners share ideas: improved mood, increased energy, sense of accomplishment, enjoyment, relaxation, etc.
4 minutes	Experience	[Do] Provide handout: **Key factors in building resilience, wellness and happiness.** [Say] To develop resilience, wellness and happiness it helps to know where to put time and effort into occupation choices. Choices based on understanding physical and mental skill that promotes adaptation and that balance self-care, productive and leisure occupations are recommended. We will read through eight key factors for building resilience as outlined by Thibeault, (2011) and Seligman, (2002).	Learners read through handout.
8 minutes	Reflection	[Say] Put a checkmark beside those key factors that you do regularly and represent an area of strength. [Ask] What is one example of an occupation you engage in that supports your area of strength?	Learners choose a minimum of one key area of personal strength. Personal response (e.g. learning creative projects supports my strength in challenging myself)

12 minutes	Generalization	[Say] Place a star * beside one key factor for resilience that you would like to develop. Name a challenge you face in developing that factor and say why it is a challenge for you.	Personal response. Examples: lack of time, money, energy, etc.
		[Do] Collect the challenges named onto the flip chart.	
		[Say] Though we may face challenges in doing some occupations for wellness, there are likely many other options we can choose. Sometimes we may forget or not take notice of things we have done to support key factors for resilience, wellness and happiness. It is also important to vary our pleasure experiences. By changing things, we continue to stimulate the pleasure centres of our brain, prevent adapting to the activities and continue to help ourselves feel good (Lyubomirsky, Sheldon & Schkade, 2005). Continue with Section 3 of the worksheet to support intentional, positive occupation choices by taking notice of wellness activities and setting goals for new experiences. Then share answers with the large group.	Learners complete the handout individually.

(continued)

Table 4.3 Cont.

Time frame	Learning stage	Facilitator	Expected learner response
15 minutes	Application	[Say] A written record of occupation choices can keep us mindful of ways we have control and responsibility to engage in occupations for resilience, wellness and happiness. [Do] Provide handout: **Occupation categories for resilience, wellness and happiness.** Invite members to complete the steps.	Learners complete the handout individually.
5 minutes	Evaluation	[Say] Choose one occupation from your handout that you would be willing to do in the next 24 hours. Share your intention with your neighbour.	Given lecture, key points for resilience, discussion, practice and feedback; The learner will construct a template for intentional positive occupation; To the extent that 2 categories to support resilience are named, each with two entry suggestions and a commitment is made to participate in one activity for happiness and wellness in the next 24 hours; As evaluated by self, peers, and therapist/facilitator.
1 minute	Wrap up	[Ask] Are there any questions? [Do] Thank everyone for coming and participating.	Personal response.

References

Layous, K., Chancellor, J., & Lyubomirsky, S. (2014). Positive activities as protective factors against mental health conditions. *Journal of Abnormal Psychology*, 123(1), 3.

Lyubomirsky, S., & Layous, K. (2013). How do simple positive activities increase well-being?. *Current Directions in Psychological Science*, 22(1), 57–62.

Lyubomirsky, S., Sheldon, K., & Schkade, D. (2005). Pursuing Happiness: The Architecture of Sustainable Change. *Review of General Psychology*. 9(2). doi.org/10.1037/1089-2680.9.2.111.

Seligman, M. E. P. (2002). *Authentic happiness: Using the new positive psychology to realize your potential for lasting fulfillment.* New York., NY: The Free Press.

Thibeault, R. (2011) Resilience and maturity. In M. A. McColl (Ed.), *Spirituality and occupational therapy.* Ottawa, ON: CAOT publications ACE.

References for Handouts

Seligman, M. E. P. (2002). *Authentic happiness: Using the new positive psychology to realize your potential for lasting fulfillment.* New York, NY: The Free Press.

Thibeault, R. (2011) Resilience and maturity. In M. A. McColl (Ed.), *Spirituality and occupational therapy.* Ottawa, ON: CAOT publications ACE.

4.4 Gratitude as Part of Daily Occupations

LEARNING POINT

Practising gratitude can improve well-being.

LEARNING OBJECTIVE

Given warm-up activity, case scenario, mix and match, worksheet, discussion, practice and feedback;

The learner will construct a gratitude journal entry;

To the extent that one written entry for each world, others and self is written, and one entry is verbally shared with the large group;

As evaluated by self, peers and therapist/facilitator.

MATERIALS

Whiteboard or flipchart and markers, labels or paper.

HANDOUTS

- Case scenario: Amara
- Sample gratitude journal: Amara
- Mix and match: Gratitude
- Mix and match: Gratitude answer sheet
- Gratitude journal

Table 4.4 Gratitude as part of daily occupations

Time frame	Learning stage	Facilitator	Expected learner response
3 minutes	Orientation	[Say] Welcome, etc. [Say] **Recognizing and expressing gratitude can increase happiness, enhance mood and improve physical well-being (Greenberger & Padesky, 2016).Gratitude involves the act of appreciating or being thankful for experiences or characteristics of the world, others and our self (Greenberger & Padesky, 2016).**	
2 minutes	Clarification	[Say] The objective is: To construct a gratitude journal entry. [Say] Today we will: • Review a case scenario with respect to gratitude • Examine benefits of expressing gratitude to self and others • Identify categories of gratitude and strategies for practice • Write a journal entry for each category of gratitude [Ask] Are we good to go?	Yes.
8 minutes	Warm-up	[Say] Think of a highlight activity for you from the last 24 hours. Write a word or draw a symbol on a label to represent that highlight. Attach it to your top.	

(*continued*)

Table 4.4 Cont.

Time frame	Learning stage	Facilitator	Expected learner response
		[Say] Introduce yourself and explain the word or symbol you chose to represent your highlight activity. Share how thinking of this highlight made you feel.	Personal response
5 minutes	Experience	[Do] Provide handout: **Case scenario: Amara** [Say] We will read this case scenario about Amara	
10 minutes	Reflection	[Ask] What were some of the negatives or hassles that Amara faced in this scenario?	Poor seating, sitting away from friend, no popcorn, etc.
		[Ask]What were some of the positives that Amara experienced?	Free night, seats available, friend available, got to see a movie she wanted, etc.
		[Ask]Were you surprised by either Amara's or her friend's reaction?	Yes or no.
		[Ask]How might you have perceived the same situation?	Personal response.
		[Ask]Have you ever had a similar experience, where you chose to focus on what you were grateful for in a situation? What impact did that have on your mood and behaviour?	Personal response.

13 minutes	Generalization	[Ask] What could be the benefits of focusing on gratitude for a situation or challenge?	You could feel better or empowered, you could continue with the task despite challenges, etc.
		[Ask] Are there any risks to focusing on gratitude for a situation or challenge?	It may take more energy and effort particularly if others in the group are being negative; making a choice to focus on gratitude keeps us responsible and accountable for our mood/ behaviour, etc.
		[Say] Practicing gratitude can strengthen positive beliefs about the world, others and our self (Greenberger & Padesky, 2016). Research shows that writing out gratitude can increase happiness scores (Seligman, 2002). Including why something makes you feel grateful in your writings has led to greater participation in exercise, less physical symptoms of anxiety, more optimism and feelings of wellness then those who recorded hassles or neutral events (Greenberger & Padesky, 2016).	

(*continued*)

Table 4.4 Cont.

Time frame	Learning stage	Facilitator	Expected learner response
		[Do] Provide handout: **Sample gratitude journal: Amara.** Read the handout out loud.	
		[Do] Provide handout: **Mix and match: Gratitude.**	
		[Say]Here are three categories of the world, others and self with a list of possible considerations for each. Match the items on the right side of the sheet with a suitable category.	Learners complete the mix and match exercise.
8 minutes	Application	[Say]There are multiple ways to practice gratitude. In groups of two or three, brainstorm ways to practice gratitude. Then share with the large group.	Write lists and post, spend time regularly contemplating gratitude, express gratitude to others, attend a weekly church service, spend time in nature reflecting on gratitude, carry a symbol as a reminder to practice gratitude, etc.
		[Do] Collect ideas on flipchart or whiteboard.	
		[Ask] Which one practice would you most likely include as part of your routine?	Personal response

| 10 minutes | Evaluation | [Do] Provide handout: **Gratitude journal**

[Say]Please complete one entry for each category on this gratitude journal. Once finished, share one entry with the large group and indicate how this practice has impacted your mood. | Given warm-up activity, case scenario, mix and match, worksheet, discussion, practice and feedback; The learner will construct a gratitude journal entry; To the extent that one written entry for each world, others and self is written, and one entry is verbally shared with the large group; As evaluated by self, peers and facilitator. |
| 1 minute | Wrap up | [Ask] Are there any questions?

[Do] Thank everyone for coming and participating. | Personal response. |

Reference

Greenberger, D., & Padesky, C. (2016). *Mind over mood: Change how you feel by changing the way you think:* (2nd ed.). New York, NY: Guilford Press.

Seligman, M. E. P. (2002). *Authentic happiness: Using the new positive psychology to realize your potential for lasting fulfillment.* New York, NY: The Free Press.

References for Handouts

Greenberger, D., & Padesky, C. (2016). *Mind over mood: Change how you feel by changing the way you think:* (2nd ed.). New York, NY: Guilford Press.

4 Change Attitude

4.1 Building On Our Strengths to Aid With Occupation Engagement

Accessing your strengths

Most of us grow from our strengths and from what we are passionate about. The questions below can help you discover your strengths. Place your answers in the spaces provided. Then, choose **one** of the options and say how it is a strength for you.

* One personal occupation in my day that I always do _____
* Something I am good at _____
* A passionate interest _____
* A subject that I know well _____
* A positive occupation I do that is valued by others _____

By focusing on our strengths and occupation successes, we can find strategies to help with challenges.

   The following process is adapted from Padesky and Mooney (2012) to build personal resilience.

1. **Find a strength**. A personal strength is discovered by answering questions such as what is one activity I always do, what is a skill I have, what positives do others say about my character, what is a subject that I know quite a lot about, what is a passionate interest I have?
2. **Identify challenges faced when engaging in my strength occupation** (e.g. feeling tired, limited time, a knowledge gap, critique from others).
3. **Identify emotions related to the named challenges** (e.g. anxiety, frustration, annoyance).
4. **Name strategies to overcome challenges**. Behaviours, thoughts and beliefs can keep us on track with the identified strength activity even when we face challenges and uncomfortable emotions. Strategies may include: I ask my friend for help, I take breaks, I say I will learn and grow if I don't give up.
5. **Choose strategies from my strength occupation to apply to other challenges** (e.g. I will ask others for help, I will take rest breaks, I will look at the challenge from a different perspective).

Reference

Padesky, C., & Mooney, K. (2012). Strengths-based cognitive-behavioural therapy: A four-step model to build resilience. *Clinical Psychology and Psychotherapy*, 19, 283–290.

Matching exercise (Max)

Max feels anxious when facing deadlines for written work reports. He identifies a personal strength occupation as: **Washing bed sheets once per week** (a "never miss" activity). Identify Max's process for using strength occupation to manage a new challenge. Match the number of the step with the described actions that follow the chart below.

Steps	Matching action
1. Identify an occupation of strength	Action D
2. Identify challenges faced with the strength occupation	
3. Identify emotions related to the challenges	
4. Strategies to stay on track with the strength occupation	
5. Conclusion: Strategies to use for other difficult occupations	

Action

A. Strategies from doing laundry that I will use for writing reports are:

- I will work in the morning when energy is higher
- I will break down big reports into smaller tasks
- I will ask my colleagues for help with tasks
- I will name a positive result from my work

B. To wash the bed sheets I:

- Do it Saturday morning when my energy is higher
- Do it in smaller steps: Wash sheet in the morning, make the bed in afternoon
- Ask others to help: My kids can strip their beds and put sheets in the wash
- Tell myself it feels good to be on clean sheets
- Remind myself I will feel better with clean sheets

C. Laundry challenges: I have other demands on my time and sometimes I am tired

D. Washing bed sheets once per week

E. Annoyed, frustration, overwhelmed

Steps in the process are adapted from Padesky & Mooney (2012).

Reference

Padesky, C., & Mooney, K. (2012). Strengths-based cognitive-behavioural therapy: A four-step model to build resilience. *Clinical Psychology and Psychotherapy*, 19, 283–290.

Using strengths to develop resilience

The following process is adapted from Padesky and Mooney (2012). They developed a model for resilience by building on those strategies we use to persevere on tasks we are passionate about, even when we face challenges.

1. Identify an occupation of strength. You may refer back to the handout: Accessing my strength:

2. Identify challenges faced with the strength occupation:

   a.

   b.

3. Identify emotions related to the challenges you named above:

4. Strategies I use to stay on track with my strength occupation, even when it is difficult:

   Behaviours:

   Thoughts:

   Beliefs:

6. Conclusion: In summary, I can use these strategies similar to those I use to keep on track with my strength occupation when challenges for other occupations occur:

   1. _____

   2. _____

   3. _____

   4. _____

Reference

Padesky, C., & Mooney, K. (2012). Strengths-based cognitive-behavioural therapy: A four-step model to build resilience. *Clinical Psychology and Psychotherapy*, 19, 283–290.

Symbol of strength

Having a symbol to represent our strengths can be a powerful reminder in new and challenging situations (Padesky & Mooney, 2012). A symbol could be an animal, book/movie character, machine, object or superhero, etc. Refer back to your strength occupation and the strategies you use even when faced with challenges. Draw a symbol to represent you and your strength occupation.

My symbol of strength

Three personal characteristics, traits or strengths associated with my symbol of strength.

1. _____

2. _____

3. _____

Now, identify a problem or occupation challenge you are facing, and briefly state why it is a challenge.

Name two strategies from the conclusion section of your worksheet: Using strengths to develop resilience, which you could apply to the occupation challenge you are facing. List them below.

1. _____

2. _____

Reference

Padesky, C., & Mooney, K. (2012). Strengths-based cognitive-behavioural therapy: A four-step model to build resilience. *Clinical Psychology and Psychotherapy*, 19, 283–290. https://doi.org/10.1002/cpp.1795.

4.2 Problem Solving to Address Challenges in Occupations

Steps to creative problem solving

1. Acknowledge the problem

The first step in solving a problem is knowing that a problem exists. Uncomfortable or distressing emotions can tell us that a problem needs to be dealt with.

2. Lay out the details of the problem

What is the problem? Why does it exist? When does it occur? Where does it occur? Who is involved?

Identify what parts are in your control and what parts of the problem are not in your control. Is there a way to restate the problem as a positive challenge or opportunity for growth?

3. Brainstorm options to manage or address the problem

All ideas are welcome at this stage as often one idea can build on another.

4. Choose options to try

Decide why an option may work for you now given your knowledge, energy, comfort level, time, finances etc.

Make a short list of one to three options to try. Decide how you will measure success.

5. Try the option

Plan how you will put your idea into practice. Include a strategy for managing challenges, discomfort or distress. Rehearse your plan and then put it into action.

6. Evaluate level of success

What went well and what was a challenge? What were you satisfied with? What did you learn from the experience? If you were to do it again, is there anything you would do differently?

What are the benefits of including all six steps?

Problem solving worksheet

1. Acknowledge the problem:

2. Lay out the details of the problem:

3. Brainstorm options to manage or address the problem (list at least three options):

4. Choose one option for trial and state your reason for the choice:
   - Option chosen:

   - My reason:

5. Try the option
   - My specific action today:

   - One resource that could help:

   - Name a positive statement that will help me take action:

   - My strategy if I get stuck or have uncomfortable emotions (circle one):

   Deep breathing   Use positive self-talk   Use humour   Talk with someone
   - Name one other coping strategy:

6. How will I evaluate my level of success with respect to my chosen option?

4.3 Intentional Positive Occupations to Boost Mental Health

Key factors in building resilience, wellness and happiness

To develop resilience, it is best to intentionally put time and effort into occupation choices that suit our needs and interests, and provide a balance of self-care, productive and leisure occupations.

Here are eight key factors in building resilience, wellness and happiness (Thibeault, 2011 and Seligman, 2002):

- Physical health – balancing our routines, self-care
- Optimism – having a belief we can succeed
- Presence – recognizing what is of value in the present moment
- Compassion – showing kindness to others and ourselves
- Challenge – taking risks, goal setting for new activity, creative projects
- Contribution – giving back through work, volunteer work, domestic activity, caregiving
- Connectedness – spending time with others that support us and bring us joy
- Gratitude – remembering to notice things and people to be grateful for

1. Place a checkmark by those factors that you do regularly. Choose a minimum of one key factor where you are strong.

2. Place a star * beside one key factor for resilience that you would like to develop.

3. It is important to notice when we choose to do occupations for resilience, wellness and happiness. It also helps to seek out new experiences that keep the pleasure centres of our brain active. *Example: I will try one new recipe on the first Sunday of each month.*

A: I will take notice of how I choose to occupy my time for resilience, wellness and happiness by:
   - Journalling
   - Scheduling my choices
   - Sharing my experiences with others
   - Daily reflection
   - Other _____

B: I will set the following goals for new experiences:

Take The Happiness Challenge:
You are invited to make a commitment to intentionally choose positive occupations for three weeks. At the end of the time period you choose, jot down two ideas of how your choices promote wellness, resilience and happiness in your life.

References

Seligman, M. E. P. (2002). *Authentic happiness: Using the new positive psychology to realize your potential for lasting fulfillment.* New York, NY: The Free Press.

Thibeault, R. (2011) Resilience and maturity. In M. A. McColl (Ed.), *Spirituality and occupational therapy.* Ottawa, ON: CAOT publications ACE.

Occupation categories for resilience, wellness and happiness

Below is a list of categories that relate to the eight key factors for boosting resilience. Choose four categories from this list that might be interesting for you or add your own idea here: _____

Physical health	Family time/ outings	Outings with partner	New Experiences
Outings with friends	Books	Movies	Treats for me
Work goals	Volunteer work	Home projects	Cleaning projects
Creative projects	New recipes	Go greener	Travel

Next, refer to the example of a journal set up below. Four categories are listed and occupation choices are identified to support the category. By structuring a journal in this fashion, we intentionally make choices for occupations we value and that promote resilience. Writing it down assists with presence, noticing our choices and remembering what we have actually done.

Example of a monthly journal set up:

Category Name	Occupation 1	Occupation 2	Occupation 3
1. Physical health	Floss once per day	30 minutes walking daily	Drink water with dinner
2. Treats for me	Walk to my favourite park	Buy a new colouring book	Take a bath
3. Try new things	New restaurant (name)	Mindfulness app	Learn a new game
4. Home projects	Clear out clutter drawer	Paint bathroom	Frame photos

Write your category choices in your journal and add occupations to support the categories, checking them off when complete.

My journal: My occupations for resilience, wellness and happiness

Category Name	Occupation 1	Occupation 2	Occupation 3
1.			
2.			
3.			
4.			

Schedule time to review your journal to recognize your choices for resilience, wellness and happiness.

4.4 Gratitude as Part of Daily Occupations

Case scenario: Amara

Amara had a last-minute cancellation for her daughter's soccer match due to bad weather. A new blockbuster movie that she wanted to see was playing at a local theatre, and now she had a free evening. She decided to call a friend and it turned out she and her daughter were also free to watch the movie.

Due to the last-minute arrangement, the only seats left available were right in the front row, causing them to sit at an awkward angle to watch the movie. In fact, her friend decided to move to another area to stand and watch the movie because she was uncomfortable. Also, the popcorn machine was broken, so neither Amara nor her friend could get the treat they promised their daughters.

At the end of the movie, Amara was happy thinking about the positives of the night's events. Her friend, however, was focusing on the negatives of the night and seemed grumpy. Amara chose to accept the negative aspects of the evening and look beyond them to acknowledge the positives of the experience. This act of gratitude shaped her mood in a positive way.

Name the negatives about Amara's situation:

Name the positives about Amara's situation:

Amara left the movie happy. Which thoughts did she choose to focus on?

(*Circle one*):   Positive thoughts   Negative thoughts

Sample gratitude journal: Amara

Recognizing and expressing gratitude can increase happiness, enhance mood and improve physical well-being (Greenberger & Padesky, 2016). Gratitude involves the act of being thankful for experiences or characteristics of the world, others and our self (Greenberger & Padesky, 2016).

World: *Things in my world that I am grateful for (e.g. community services, diversity)*
Others: *Others that I am grateful for (e.g. family, friends, coworkers, pets)*
Self: *Things about myself that I am grateful for (e.g. qualities, strengths, kind acts)*

The following is a sample from Amara's gratitude journal.

World: I live in a neighbourhood where I feel safe to walk to activities, including a local movie theatre. Many faces in my neighbourhood are familiar to me and people are friendly.

Others: I have several close friends who share my interests and are glad to hear from me, even if it is for a last-minute request. My daughter and I enjoy laughing together.

Self: I enjoy being spontaneous. I felt happy that we went to a movie to distract from the disappointment of her game being cancelled. I taught her an important lesson of not dwelling on the negatives and finding new opportunities.

Reference

Greenberger, D., & Padesky, C. (2016). *Mind over mood: Change how you feel by changing the way you think*: (2nd ed.). New York, NY: Guilford Press.

Mix and match: Gratitude
Match the category on the left to the items on the right

World

I thanked the grocery clerk for doing a great job packing my groceries.

I live in a country where we experience freedoms in speech, religious worship and cultural practices.

I have a pet that is always happy to see me and loves to spend time with me.

I am part of a community that values healthy lifestyles, and the politicians advocate for safer roads for cyclists, traffic calming measures and local programs for seniors.

Others

I am interested in being friendly to others and say hello to others as I pass them on the street.

I have a good sense of humour.

A friend knew I was having a hard time and offered to come and spend some time with me.

I called a person who was a role model to me in the past and thanked him for his mentorship.

Self

My co-worker thanked me for my efforts in dealing with a challenging situation today.

My family makes an effort to stay in touch and see each other several times a year.

Mix and match: Gratitude answer sheet

World

I live in a country where we experience freedoms in speech, religious worship and cultural practices.

I am part of a community that values healthy lifestyles, and the politicians advocate for safer roads for cyclists, traffic calming measures and local programs for seniors.

Others

I have a pet that is always happy to see me and loves to spend time with me.

A friend knew I was having a hard time and offered to come and spend some time with me.

My co-worker thanked me for my efforts in dealing with a challenging situation today.

My family makes an effort to stay in touch and see each other several times a year.

Self

I thanked the grocery clerk for doing a great job packing my groceries.

I am interested in being friendly to others and say hello to others as I pass them on the street.

I have a good sense of humour.

I called a person who was a role model to me in the past and thanked him.

Gratitude journal

Gratitude journals are a way of changing your mindset to a more positive mindset. By feeling grateful, it gives you different thoughts about the world, others or self. Feel free to be creative. Over time, this journal will become a story and record of your feelings and warm experiences of what you have given, and also what you have received. You can always look back at it as a reminder of what brings you happiness.

Date: _____

Today I am grateful for ...

1. *World: Things in my world that I am grateful for:*

2. *Others: Things about family, friends, coworkers, pets, supports that I am grateful for:*

3. *Self: Qualities, strengths, acts of kindness, about myself that I am grateful for:*

By choosing to focus on gratitude, I am boosting my mood and well-being!

Index